The Making of Rehabilitation

Steve Sturdy

Wellcome Unit for the
History of Medicine

Manchester University

Feb. 1990.

The Making of Rehabilitation

A Political Economy of Medical Specialization, 1890–1980

Glenn Gritzer
and
Arnold Arluke

UNIVERSITY OF CALIFORNIA PRESS

Berkeley • *Los Angeles* • *London*

University of California Press
Berkeley and Los Angeles, California

University of California Press, Ltd.
London, England

Library of Congress Cataloging in Publication Data

Gritzer, Glenn.
The making of rehabilitation medicine.

  (Comparative studies of health systems and
medical care)
    Includes index.
    1. Rehabilitation—Political aspects—History—
19th century.   2. Rehabilitation—Political aspects—
United States—History—19th century.   3. Rehabilitation
—Political aspects—History—20th century.   4. Rehabilitation—Political aspects—United States—History—
20th century.   5. Rehabilitation—Economic aspects—
History—19th century.   6. Rehabilitation—Economic
aspects—United States—History—19th century.
7. Rehabilitation—Economic aspects—History—20th
century.   8. Rehabilitation—Economic aspects—
United States—History—20th century.   I. Arluke, Arnold.
II. Title. III. Series. [DNLM: 1. Occupational Therapy
—history—United States.   2. Physical Medicine—history
—United States.   3. Physical Therapy—history—
United States.   4. Rehabilitation—history—United States.
WZ 70 AA1 G68m]
RM930.G75   1985   362.1'786'0973   84-28008
ISBN 0-520-05302-8

Printed in the United States of America

1 2 3 4 5 6 7 8 9

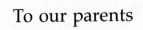

To our parents

Contents

FOREWORD   xi

ACKNOWLEDGMENTS   xxiii

1
Introduction   1

    The Natural Growth Model   2
    The Market Model   7
    Rehabilitation Medicine   11

2
The Bases for Specialization, 1890–1917   15

    Electricity: A Base for Organization   17
        Early Champions of Electricity   17
        Physicians Organize   20
    Enlarging the Base   26
        Internal Competition   26
        External Competition   32
    The Response to AMA Rejection   34

3
War and the Organization of Work, 1917–1920   38

    The War Wounded and Occupational
    Conflict   39
        Internal Competition   39
        External Conflict   46

The Origins of the Allied Occupations   52
    Physical Therapy   52
    Occupational Therapy   54
    The Impact of War   57

4
Foundations for a Division of Labor, 1920–1941   61

    Physical Therapy Physicians Between
    the Wars   62
        Professional Developments   62
        The Battle Against Competitors   64
    The Allied Occupations:
    Institutionalization and Subordination   70
        Physical Therapy   70
        Occupational Therapy   78

5
The Rediscovery of Rehabilitation, 1941–1950   86

    World War II and Physical Medicine   87
        The Influence of "Outsiders"   91
        Expansion and a New Name   94
    Allied Occupations in the War   99
        Physical Therapy   99
        Occupational Therapy   104
    Early Postwar Years   108
        The Veterans Administration   109
        The Physical Medicine and
        Rehabilitation Service   111
        The Allied Occupations   114
    Physical Medicine and Rehabilitation
    at Midcentury   118

6
The Redivision of Labor, 1950–1980   123

    Pursuit of Autonomy   124
        The Rise of Physical Therapy   124
        Occupational Therapy's Market
        Mistakes   135

The Fall from Power   145
   Marginality and Supply Problems   145
   Market Challenges   148

Epilogue   159

The Bases for Rigidity and
Imperialism   161

APPENDIXES   171
  A. Changes in Occupational Titles   173
  B. Professional Associations and
     Journals: Physicians   174
  C. Professional Associations and
     Journals: Allied Occupations   176

NOTES   177

INDEX   207

Foreword

Eliot Freidson

The division of labor represents two of the most fundamental characteristics that mark human life off from that of other animals—the capacity to create tools that aid in the performance of specialized tasks, and the capacity to cooperate with others in the performance of complementary tasks that yield a joint product. It exists in some form in every human society, but wherever society is complex and reasonably large it is composed in large degree of formally defined, stable occupations in which workers specialize in various tasks that produce the goods and services on which human life depends. The division of labor is thus the *generic* basis for differentiation in human life. While it is possible to imagine a society undivided by class inequality, we cannot imagine a viable society undivided by specialization. And if we wish to imagine a society with a rich material and cultural standard of living, we could not imagine one without a fairly stable structure of differentiation by specialization.

As fundamental as is the division of labor in the human scheme of things, it has not been the focus for much thought and study. Of the classic writers, Durkheim provides us with the idea that the number of different specializations in a division of labor can be explored as a function of size and density of population, but that idea does not allow us to understand why the particular specializations arise in the first place and why they assume the form they do. Adam Smith considered its growth to be a critical prerequisite for increased productivity and "universal opulence," but did not address it directly as a topic for analysis. His comments on "combinations" and mercantilism were, as usual, shrewd, and his emphasis on the role of self-interest and competition in the offering and consumption of goods and services in the free market provides us with one set of possible tools by which the development and maintenance of a particular division of labor can be traced. But his emphasis on an ideal free market prevented him from developing concepts capable of dealing with the way real markets are actually constituted and operated. And while Karl Marx did suggest a rudimentary typology of various ways in which divisions of labor may be organized, his primary focus was on the detailed division of labor of the industrial enterprises of his time, the concept of division of labor remaining vague and contradictory in his work. Obsessed with capital and its role in creating the basic order of industrial society, Marx provided some understanding of why the detailed division of labor developed in factories but little or no understanding of how or why the particular social division of labor of a given time and place and even any particular detailed division of labor in a given factory develops, maintains itself, and changes. Classic theorists thus give us only modest help.

In order to understand the division of labor better, it seems clear that some basic facts must be taken into account. Above all, it is essential to recognize that divisions of labor are socially organized. One cannot merely add up all specialized occupations or jobs into a sum and declare that to be the division of labor. After all, insofar as they are specialized, occupations are interdependent and thus must have socially organized relations with one another. In one way or another specialized tasks must be coordinated for some common outcome. A number of jobs in a given enterprise, then, must be part of a coordinating social organization. That coordinating social organization, however, is clearly a historic variable and not a universal constant: just as there is more than one way to skin a cat, so there is more than one way to organize a division of labor.

Similarly, the elements constituting the division of labor—the particular assortment of individual tasks that gets collected into a job or work role—may not be thought to be constants. While there are certainly spatial, temporal, and material limits to the number and variety of tasks that possibly can be performed by an individual worker, and while there are certainly other purely mechanical or technological constraints, there is nonetheless a broad area of indeterminacy which allows a number of possible combinations of various tasks to be crystallized into the social role bundles we call jobs, occupations, trades, or specialties. The question is, what is the process by which those bundles are made up and by which they are organized into a functioning social system? Who are the effective actors in that process, what powers do they exercise and how do they exercise them? These are some of the questions we must answer if we are to gain a better understanding of the division of labor.

At present we have only the crudest of tools with which to fashion a theory by which we can guide our efforts at answering such questions. In the face of the obvious fact that divisions of labor can be constituted and organized by different social agents, we can invoke the accepted distinction between bureaucratic and craft, or administrative and occupational, principles of organization. The bureaucratic or administrative method invokes the monocratic exercise of economic and political power to create and control a rational-legal system of formulating, organizing, and controlling the work which people do in public and private firms. In that case the division of labor is a creation of the management of the firm, and serves the interests of its owners more directly than it does the interests of those who do the productive work. The jobs in such a division of labor are in theory formulated as precisely and simply as possible so that supervision and control are facilitated. Supervision, control, and the very division of labor itself are organized hierarchically.

As a model, this bureaucratic concept of Max Weber's does not reflect the wide empirical deviations that exist in the real world, but it does help us conceive of the way the division of labor is created and organized in the vast majority of large firms of both capitalist and state socialist industrial nations. Neither the particular jobs of the division of labor nor the coordinative organization of their interrelations are created by those who perform them. Rather, the jobs are created by others in order to serve the ends of investors or the Party. And understandably enough, those who fill such jobs in such hierarchically structured divisions of labor sometimes lack the enthusiasm which their superordinates would like. They are objectively alienated by virtue of their relation to their jobs and subjectively alienated by virtue of their response to that relation.

This bureaucratic or administrative principle for developing, organizing, and controlling a division of labor has been studied and discussed extensively by business management and organizational theorists. It is marked by the assertive and controlling role of managers and the passive role of workers. In contrast, the craft or occupational principle for organizing work has been studied and discussed far less but, when it has been, it marks active attempts at control on the part of the workers themselves, who form occupational groups and negotiate the substance and shape of the division of labor. One historic version of that method is to be found in the guilds of an earlier day, another in the organized crafts today, and still another, of far greater theoretical and practical importance, is to be found in the rapidly growing professional-technical segment of the labor force. A particular group of workers becomes joined together around a common occupational title and attempts to gain more or less exclusive right both to the title and to the right to specialize in the performance of a specific set of tasks associated with it. Only professional and sometimes technical workers today, along with those in the crafts, have the capacity to organize what Max Weber called "social closures," or shelters, in the labor market that protect their titles and their job rights. All others, including managers and administrators themselves, are almost wholly at the mercy of the policies of the particular public or private firms that employ them.

Since specialization presupposes interdependence, part of the process of establishing the boundaries of a specialty inevitably requires negotiation among contiguous occupational groups over the lines demarcating their efforts one from the other. And since coordination of interdependent efforts is essential, part of the negotiation must deal with the issue of responsibility and control. Will the division of labor among interdependent occupations be coordinated by the collective judgment of the participants as the flow of work proceeds, or will there be key occupations whose members are responsible for coordinating and controlling the efforts of others? The issues of jurisdiction—that is, the particular tasks claimed by the members of a particular occupation—and of control have been especially problematic in the creation of occupational methods of constituting divisions of labor simply because the method itself, unlike the bureaucratic or administrative method, presupposes no hierarchical authority that has the legitimate right to determine them. Thus, a great deal more overt competition and conflict is likely to be evident in the formation of an occupationally controlled division of labor than in an administratively controlled system.

Gritzer and Arluke's book may be taken as a case study of the process by which an occupationally controlled division of labor was formed. It provides us with a detailed view of how the people now providing what are known as rehabilitation services came to be organized into particular occupations with limited jurisdictions and specific positions in the health division of labor mandated by public or private law. It is thus a history of the development of a formal division of labor, the structure of which is stabilized through the creation of social closures, or shelters, in the labor market. The characteristic method employed by occupations in the general area of health care, though less common in other areas, is to seek legally enforced shelters through state licensing or the establishment of standards for staffing jobs that require specific credentials.

Beginning with physicians who took up the technology of electrotherapy as a specialty in the late nineteenth century, this book traces the vicissitudes of their attempts to establish a secure position in the medical marketplace, first as electrotherapists and then as physiotherapists. The security of such a position depended on the recognition and acceptance of other physicians: willingness not to treat patients themselves, but instead refer them to a specialist, can make the difference between success and failure. Related to recognition and acceptance by other physicians is the issue of excluding potential competitors from practice—something that requires political action on the part of an organized group. And if not exclusion from competition entirely, negotiation can lead to subordinating potential competitive practice by putting it in a place in the division of labor where it is subject to the supervision and control of physicians. The American Medical Association, representing practitioners, and the American Hospital Association, representing employers, were key agents in the process of political negotiation that shaped the division of labor that emerged—a division of labor constituted by a particular set of occupations (many of whose names or titles changed over time) and structured by both referral and supervisory relations.

This is not the place to deal with the details of the process by which that particular division of labor emerged. That, after all, is what the book does. Nor is it the place to discuss the complexity of the relations between medical specialties, nonmedical occupations that have found a subordinate niche in the medically controlled segment of the health division of labor, and nonmedical occupations that stand outside it and act as real or potential competitors to those inside. Instead, let me comment briefly on several important themes in Gritzer and Arluke's book.

One theme is the role of the state in the formation and maintenance of the division of labor in general and the division of labor in the professional trades in particular. That topic has been seriously neglected in the American literature, for most of it has been created in the context of the special circumstances of the United States where the role of the state has not been conspicuous until very recently. But even in the United States the state has always provided the foundation for establishing and sustaining divisions of labor. The powers which employers have to create and control the jobs that constitute the division of labor in their firms rest on legally defined rights of property-owners. Even labor law designed to provide workers with rights to organize and negotiate with employers reserves to management rights to define and supervise the division of labor.

An even more obvious role is played by the state in those instances where the division of labor is controlled by occupations. While firms exercise control through the constitution of their own internal labor markets, occupations have to develop methods of carving out a social closure or shelter in the general or external labor market from which labor consumers seek workers. A conspicuous method by which this is done relies on occupational licensing, a method that requires the support of law and therefore of the state. Licensing attempts to establish the boundaries of the bundles of tasks that may be performed exclusively by a given occupation, and if that occupation can also restrict entry so as to keep supply adjusted to demand, then its economic security is assured. Licensing is especially conspicuous in the field of health, where arguments of protecting the public are especially persuasive, and there it sustains the position of occupations like medicine and dentistry and also establishes the subordination of occupations like nursing and dental hygiene to their "superior" occupations in the division of labor.

The importance of licensing has been exaggerated, however. Far more important in the United States is a less conspicuous system whereby the state does not itself create labor market shelters by licensing but rather adopts and ratifies the procedures and criteria for qualification created by private professional associations and the associations representing both educational (that is, credential-producing) institutions and those employing professionals. Thus, the many private "specialty boards" in medicine are all recognized by both the federal government and the states, as are a variety of forms of accreditation of professional institutions and certification of professionals. Such recognition is not very important unless significant benefits are attached to it, however, and there is where the role of the state in influencing the substance and organization of the professional division of labor has been changing rapidly since World War II, particularly in the field of health.

Since the federal government has taken to paying for some of the health care bills of patients, it must decide which are legitimate to reimburse and which are not, and what kinds of credentials attest to the legitimacy of those providing services. This means that even self-employed practitioners develop an economic stake in possessing the credentials that the state recognizes. However, the vast majority of all professions and professionals in the United States is typically employed. It is for this reason that the greatest impact of the state on the division of labor is to be found in its capacity to create and sustain specialized jobs in its own agencies, and to specify the credentials necessary for jobs in private institutions that require its approval and support.

Gritzer and Arluke's study is very clear about the importance of the state in the development of the division of labor in the rehabilitation services. The two World Wars vastly expanded the market for such services, and they presented opportunities for the creation of new specialties and the expansion of established specialties. Furthermore, facilities to provide services to veterans continued after hostilities ceased, so that after each war jobs for rehabilitation occupations continued to be provided by the state. The struggle among contending occupations and specialties was over whose credentials would be chosen for the jobs, who would have commissioned rank in the armed forces, and which occupation would be in control of the relevant division of labor. The choices that were made during mobilization lived on in the postwar period, only slowly changing in the course of later events.

When the federal government began to finance civilian health care expenditures in the 1960s, however, the role of the state extended far beyond that of being an employer, which was the case in wartime and in postwar veterans' facilities. In reimbursing for health services provided by self-employed practitioners, it had to settle on criteria by which it could determine the legitimacy of claims. Its choices had critical economic importance for occupations offering services, and were the focus of the political activities of the professional associations representing them. For the occupations engaged in providing services related to rehabilitation, however, by far the most important role of the state was in determining the criteria that would justify reimbursing the claims of health care organizations like hospitals. In that instance the issue becomes institutional staffing—what occupations, with what titles and credentials, should be employed by the institution to provide the services for which the state is billed. There too we find complex lobbying efforts on the part of professional associations seeking to gain exclusive recognition of their own and those allied with them, and to defeat the efforts of other occupations to gain recognition. The prize thus created is the virtual requirement imposed by the state on employing organizations like hospitals that certain jobs will be filled only by those with certain credentials on pain of losing the right to reimbursement. In the struggle among occupations and between occupations and organizational managers to establish the content and structure of the division of labor, then, the state can become a critical arbiter even when it does not have the direct power to command the division of labor. Gritzer and Arluke provide plenty of grist for those who wish to explore that relationship more deeply.

Another issue raised by Gritzer and Arluke is at the core of their general argument—namely, the role of technology, scientific knowledge, and skill in determining the direction of the development of new techniques and specialized occupations in the division of labor. They provide details in their history which allow laying the ghost of technological determinism in explaining the specializations that emerged in the division of labor in the field of rehabilitation. They show that it could easily have been otherwise. One may lay the ghost of crude technological determinism, however, and still not destroy the value of the idea that available knowledge, skill, and technology do place limits on the variety and type of specialties that develop in any given time and on the exact substance of the division of labor.

One may think with some justice that the aim or goal of work places some limits on what work will be done and how it will be organized. While there is more than one way to skin a cat, if the aim is to skin a cat, there are only a limited number of possible ways of choosing, dividing up, and performing the tasks of doing so. If, on one hand, an aim is very concrete and limited, then the possibilities for variation must also be limited. If, on the other hand, it is poorly delineated, vague, and shifting, the possibility for variation in the tasks to be performed and in the organization of task performance into division of labor is much greater.

"Rehabilitation" is a vague and poorly delineated concept, and its concrete aims subject to a fair degree of variation. It has included physical training as well as vocational education, concrete surgical repair and correction as well as psychotherapy. Given such a variety of procedures connected with the overall field, one should expect many kinds of occupations to have a potential contribution to make, and thus a fairly large number of possibilities for constituting a division of labor. It would improve our understanding of the process by which a division of labor is constituted and sustained if we were to replicate the Gritzer and Arluke study in other health fields, and most particularly fields whose aims are more determinate and concrete. A history of the division of labor in surgery, for example, would be a useful comparison. I suspect that it would certainly show some of the same arbitrariness in the formation of specialties and their domains and in the distribution of specific tasks that Gritzer and Arluke uncover. Nonetheless, I suspect also that variation in the division of labor and in the agents empowered to control and coordinate it would operate within narrower limits than was the case for rehabilitation, and would show a certain technical logic that is much more difficult to find in rehabilitation. But that is speculation on my part and I may very well be wrong. Gritzer and Arluke's study fairly begs for others in the same tradition that would begin to allow systematic comparisons. Comparative analysis is essential for developing a more sophisticated and better grounded conception of the limits that knowledge and technique impose on specialization and the division of labor.

Finally, I wish to comment on the issue of interpreting the motives of members of occupational groups which is raised by Gritzer and Arluke's study and most other studies that adopt a "market approach" to the analysis of occupations. The emphasis of such an approach is on how members of an occupation manage to gain a reasonably steady living from it, an emphasis that is entirely justified by the fact that without a living its members are unlikely to continue to work at that occupation and the occupation is therefore unlikely to survive. The survival of occupations depends upon establishing a viable place in the labor market.

The market approach is without doubt an indispensable element of analysis. Its danger, however, is that by its selective emphasis it gives the impression that members of the occupation are motivated primarily by material self-interest and that their efforts to extend the application of their skills to new fields are fueled primarily by the desire to improve their own position in the labor market, or to expand the number of available jobs so as to expand the ranks of the occupation for the sake of expansion alone. Plausible as the idea of material self-interest is to our twentieth-century Anglo-American minds, it constitutes only a partial and highly selective characterization of the complexity of human activity. It is best fitted to analyze something that has never existed in reality—namely, the totally fluid conditions of a truly free market. In present-day reality, it is probably best fitted to the circumstances of casual labor—those who are physically, psychologically, and socially free of all other commitments but income and who can therefore shift from one kind of work to another solely on the basis of maximizing income. In contrast, the idea of material self-interest is probably least fitted to members of occupations who have become committed not only to their occupations as a source of income but also to the work itself. Well-organized occupations like the professions and the crafts are characterized by such commitment to "intrinsic" as well as "extrinsic" rewards, as are those special and poorly organized occupations surrounding the arts whose behavior Adam Smith ascribed to overweening conceit rather than to rational self-interest, and whose Bohemian status Marx assigned to the Lumpenproletariat.

One cannot read the documents left by past members of such occupations without having to recognize commitment to and concern with their work. Nor can one interview contemporary members without recognizing frequent expressions of interest in the work itself and genuine belief in its value and importance. Claims for the work certainly can function to advance the economic fortunes of the occupation and its members, and they may be made consciously to serve the end of economic advancement, but they are likely to be believed by those who advance them. The motives for advancing them cannot be exhausted by imputing economic self-interest and status-striving alone. Self-interest is in interaction with commitment to the occupation, its particular set of tasks or techniques, its characteristic work-relations and work-settings. While the market approach to the study of the professions has been invaluable in clearing away some of the pious ideological fog surrounding them in past work and in revealing their economic foundation, it needs to be integrated into a more subtle and complex framework that includes attention to the very real effects of noneconomic motives—cognitive as well as noncognitive—in establishing, advancing, and changing the work of occupations and their place in the division of labor. Gritzer and Arluke's book takes the first step of analyzing the markets involved. Let us hope that they or others will take the next.

Acknowledgments

Much of this book was prepared under predoctoral grants from the United States Public Health Service No. HS 00013, and the Commonwealth Foundation Program in Law, Science and Medicine at Yale Law School. Support provided by DHHS grant No. RR07143, and the Provost's Research and Development Fund of Northeastern University made it possible to undertake substantial revisions of early drafts.

Our primary intellectual debt is to Eliot Freidson whose thinking about professions supplied the starting point and focus for this project. We also thank Wolf Heydebrand, Herbert Menzel, Peter New, Julius Roth, and Phyllis Stewart for helpful comments at various stages of the manuscript's development. As series editor, Charles Leslie offered valuable guidance in reshaping the manuscript and patience with the authors' often slow progress. Others were vitally helpful along the way in their support for the project, including Adrea Barry, Karen Jacobsen, Elliott Krause, and Jack Levin. Finally, we would like to thank Flora Hollins, Marilyn Churchill, and Marc Fisher for typing the manuscript.

1

Introduction

This century has witnessed an explosion of specialties in the health care field. When the United States entered World War I, one medical specialty was recognized by the American Medical Association (AMA). A handful of other specialties were organized by the 1930s but attracted only 17 percent of all physicians to full-time specialty practice. At present, fifty-two specialties are recognized by the AMA and approximately 80 percent of all physicians are specialists. Moreover, almost every medical specialty has one or more recognized subspecialties. Psychiatry, for example, has subspecialties in social psychiatry, forensic psychiatry, psychopharmacology, and family therapy. Some subspecialties have divided even further. Within hematology, a subspecialty of internal medicine, there are at least four types of hematologists.[1]

The specialty picture in the health care field appears even more complex when one considers the variety of allied health personnel, or nonphysician practitioners, that now exist. In 1910 the health care "team" consisted of three members—physicians, nurses, and aides. By the 1970s well over 500 allied health care occupations had arisen.[2] Many of these specialties, like their physician counterparts, have created subspecialties.

1

In nursing, for example, there are specialties in geriatrics, pediatrics, and psychiatry, to name only a few. Some allied health occupations have also created new kinds of workers at the assistant or technician level. In addition to considering the sheer number of individual specialties, a proper view of the current state of specialization in the health care field must consider the kinds of relationships that exist among specialties. The latter is addressed by the concept of the division of labor, a concept that presupposes some set of mechanisms ordering the interrelationships of specialties.[3] In the health care field these mechanisms are thought to be necessary to provide patient care in a coordinated, nonfragmented manner by different specialties.

Yet anxieties have grown in recent years over the undesirable effects of "overspecialization" on the quality of patient care and the inability of the medical division of labor to coordinate the work of the many specialties. Critics charge that there is little communication among and between specialties and even less coherent communication with the patient. It is argued that individual specialists, if they yield to other specialists at all, do so only when boundaries of expertise have been reached. Indeed, it is evident to one commentator "that boundary walls are being built ever higher around separate and antagonistic identities."[4] These anxieties have led to simplistic calls for "teamwork" or "collegial relationships" in medicine rather than any systematic analysis of the underlying forces that explain why specialization occurs and how a division of labor is constructed.

The Natural Growth Model

Why has the practice of medicine become so specialized and its division of labor so complex? The most popular, but too facile, explanation is that specialization is a natural and inevitable consequence of scientific progress. According to this argument, divisions of medical work are directly determined by technological innovation and growth in knowledge. Medical historian Stanley Reiser finds that specialization is "stimulated by the multiplication of scientific instruments" and the "absolute increase in medical knowledge."[5] Physician Richard Macgraw asserts that the process of specialization "is natural, irresistible, and shows no sign of slackening. Informal and de facto subspecialization within these fields constantly develops as a natural extension of new knowledge and new techniques."[6] In this view technology and knowledge have a life of their own, and impose their own imperatives on the organization of work.

This natural growth model of specialization is often accepted at face value; it forms part of our modern view about the necessary forms for organizing work in a scientific age. Constant references are made, for example, to the "knowledge explosion" outstripping the capacity of any one practitioner to master an entire field.[7] In these discussions, specialization is seen as an essential component of work in the twentieth century. Beyond mere necessity, the specialist is even glorified as the symbol of our progress and our times. It is not surprising that the need in a complex society for a division of labor and for specialists is taken for granted, and the actual division of labor that develops in particular fields is regarded as unproblematic.

The natural growth model is an integral part of contemporary thinking about the organization of work because it is deeply rooted in Western social thought. In the eighteenth and nineteenth centuries ideas of progress and evolution emerged to explain social change. These notions emphasized the potential for unlimited development as opposed to earlier views of human capacity and morality, which were cyclical and generally more pessimistic.[8] According to historians Kenneth Bock and Frederick Taggart, the ideas of progress and evolution, although new to the industrial age, were based on a biological analogy inherent in the intellectual tradition of Western cultures.[9] Social change and development of the individual organism were seen in the same way—necessary, immanent, purposive, directional, cumulative, irreversible, and occurring in stages. Similarly, sociologist Robert Nisbet traces the concepts of progress and evolution to a Western mode of thought he calls the natural growth metaphor. The concept of the natural, as that which unfolds in an immanent fashion according to laws, excluded accidental or unique occurrences and thus excluded history from the new scientific study of society in general, and from the notions of progress and evolution in particular.[10]

To deal with changes in the nature of work brought about by the Industrial Revolution, social theorists of that era created the concept of the division of labor based on natural growth, progress, and evolution.[11] They argued that technology, science, population pressure, and human striving for improvement led inexorably to greater work differentiation, and that specialization and functional interdependence were the automatic and unplanned foundations of the new society. The key questions for these utilitarians were not division of labor by whom, in what manner, or for what particular reason. They used the concept to disguise the role of power-based relationships in the organization of work, and to argue against interference in the workings of natural processes.[12]

Émile Durkheim further developed this tradition in his book *The Division of Labor in Society*, in which he investigated the evolving basis of social solidarity.[13] He held the utilitarian view that differentiation was an automatic process derived from ecological forces. However, he challenged the view that functional interdependence based on the "natural identity of individual interests" would be the basis for the new society. He recast the concept by arguing that the shared beliefs and moral rules socially generated in a new division of labor would serve this purpose. Durkheim's concern was to study this new moral basis rather than to analyze the organization of work.[14]

Durkheim questioned the fate of individuals and society when economic interests became key points for social interaction, but he resolved questions about conflicts between labor and the owners of capital by defining them as "abnormal" forms of an essentially "healthy" new division of labor. He ignored the importance of class conflict in determining the division of labor and the overall form of the new industrial society. Durkheim assumed automatic processes of differen-

tiation and interdependence, and continued a sterile, apo-
litical conceptualization of division of labor. The concept thus
served to obscure how work was organized, specifically the
struggle to control skill and the labor process.

Modern social thinkers have continued to ground the division of labor concept in the natural growth metaphor. Prior
to the 1970s the sociological study of occupations was rooted
in this metaphor. The attribute approach to the study of
professions shared the assumptions that inexorable forces result in automatic specialization and reintegration of work, that
inherent characteristics determine professional development,
and that these traits set professions apart from other occupations. These assumptions led sociologists to ignore the social organization of work and to focus instead on enumerating
the special attributes of professions. Also, this perspective
treated power as derived from rather than as the basis for
these attributes.

The work of the sociologist William Goode best illustrates
this approach to the professions. In the 1960s Goode focused
on two core attributes determining professional status: "pro-
longed specialized training in a body of abstract knowledge,
and a collectivity or service orientation."[15] Focusing on these
attributes, Goode ignored questions about occupational specialization and coordination. The attribute of special knowledge accounted for differentiation and stratification of work
roles; parameters of knowledge plus the claimed service orientation sustained belief in automatic interdependence. For
Goode, all other variables, such as power, autonomy, and
status, were determined by the two core attributes.

The assumed link between knowledge and occupational
specialization usually remained implicit in his analysis, the
problem having been defined out of existence. On one occasion, however, Goode articulated this connection, stating
that an "occupation may, as its knowledge base grows, simply
split into numerous subassociations." He also noted that "the
rapid growth of knowledge and its organization into specialties encourages each subgroup to focus on its own interests."[16]

The persistence of the natural growth metaphor stems from

its ideological function of ascribing spontaneous growth and development to particular historical events. The decision about which events are natural and immanently unfolding and which are accidental becomes an evaluative choice that merges what ought to be and what is in a single line of development. Thus Thomas Kuhn's description of "scientific revolutions" showed how major changes lead to the recasting of previous work to make it consistent with currently dominant "paradigms." Scientist-historians reinterpret these "revolutions" by selecting those discoveries that fit into a framework of linear development. As Kuhn says, "the deprecation of historical fact is deeply, and probably functionally, ingrained in the ideology of the scientific profession."[17]

A similar relativistic stance was developed earlier by German historicists and carried on by Karl Marx. It was largely those inspired by the Marxian tradition who unmasked the vested interests, power, and conflict concealed in the capitalist view of progress. An example of this critique is the work of Georges Sorel, who demonstrated that dominant groups use the idea of progress to legitimate their power by depicting the past as necessarily leading to a present state of enlightenment, and by projecting the immanent unfolding of knowledge and moral perfection into the future.[18]

For Nisbet, the natural growth metaphor persists since it is "integrative in its social and psychological effects upon groups."[19] He points to nationalistic groups which interpret past events as prophetic signs in their movement's development. A similar use of the metaphor by occupational groups makes it necessary to treat their historical accounts as little more than self-serving ideological statements. Histories written by practitioners typically describe the development of their occupations as a continuous process spurred by cumulative knowledge growth. They portray their occupations as having "emerged" and "evolved" to their present state. Clearly, this "rhetoric of evolution" will continue to be affirmed by some, and believed by many, until attention is paid to the generic phenomenon of specialization and the forces that determine the division of labor.[20] To do this requires an entirely different approach to the organization of work.

The Market Model

We need not accept the inevitability of specialization; its mere existence fails to explain why specialties develop and how a division of labor is constructed. If the division of labor is to be treated as a subject requiring explanation, rather than as a given due to advances in knowledge and technology, a model logically and substantively in contrast to the natural growth model is needed. This book develops such an alternative approach.

The market model of specialization is suggested in the recent work of sociologists and others concerned with the rise of the medical profession in nineteenth- and twentieth-century America.[21] These researchers have started to explore an approach that focuses on the ways in which an occupation, as an organized body of workers, establishes a secure and successful position in the political economy by seeking to control the supply of, and demand for, their services. From this perspective, specialization and coordination of work must be seen as intimately intertwined with, and an outgrowth of, the struggle among occupations to organize markets by gaining the exclusive right to exercise certain skills and to perform certain tasks. Rather than causing specialization, knowledge and technology can be resources used by interested groups to justify specialty status and dominance in a division of labor.

Occupational groups coalesce, according to sociologist Magali Sarfatti Larson, when groups of workers organize markets for their services.[22] The first task in constituting and controlling their markets is to make their "product" or service recognizable and identifiable to consumers. For Larson, such commodity definition is achieved after the group acquires an esoteric body of knowledge, sufficiently uniform and standard to permit the training of practitioners in that field. Once such a cognitive base is formed, an occupational organization can develop.

However, significant commodity definition needs to occur prior to attaining a cognitive base.[23] Initial organization of workers requires that those providing similar services recognize their shared expertise and interests. Similarly, consumers must recognize the commodity to establish the economic viability of the service. Both organization and economic resources, in turn, are necessary to pursue the "professional project"—elaboration of a uniquely possessed cognitive base transmitted to trainees in an educational setting controlled by the occupational group.

For medical specialties, the cognitive dimension develops later in the game and is the outcome of occupational organization rather than its cause or the vehicle for its occurrence. What is critical to specialty formation is the simple and concrete, not the complex or esoteric. Material factors such as technologies define a sphere of work to insiders and outsiders. Physicians who specialize in their use develop uniquely held skills in the actual application of the technology and empirical observations about its clinical effects. Practitioners often characterize technical or manual skills as more critical and much early attention is devoted to improving skill in applying rudimentary devices.

These initial bases for specialty formation are distinctly different from customary assumptions about specialization. Technical skills in utilizing mechanical devices are usually accepted as the bases for craft occupations but not for professional groups. The development of clinical expertise and judgment is closer to our accustomed notions about the work that "professionals" perform. Virtually absent, however, is a recognizable body of theoretical knowledge whose mastery could be claimed to require specialization. Rather, specialty groups may form around service "commodities" defined by readily recognizable technical devices. Later, in their struggles to secure the market for their services, claimed theoretical knowledge becomes an important component in the professional project.

The development of medical specialties also depends on the ability of groups of workers to take advantage of unique historical events. This notion is contrary to the natural growth model, which treats the process of specialization in a social and political vacuum. Events such as war, for example, provide special opportunities to groups having a low status because of their involvement in activities previously outside regular medicine. Marginal or nascent medical groups may engage in tactics aimed at upward mobility and recognition by the medical profession. In particular, they may try to improve their position by meeting the rapid escalation of wartime demand for health care and by demonstrating the efficacy of their techniques. Regular physicians may be persuaded to use these techniques and, in so doing, grant these techniques a degree of legitimacy they previously lacked. In this stage of the development of a specialty, the market strategy is to court the medical profession and not claim exclusive competence. Gaining the profession's acceptance improves commodity definition and enlists the power of the profession in combating nonphysician competitors in the open market.

History also plays a crucial role in the development of allied occupations. The expansion of a subordinate division of labor may begin with sudden heightened demand for medical services during wartime. Physicians, unable to meet this demand completely, may provide active assistance in forming and promoting allied occupations. Tasks that are unpleasant, or lack esteem, such as the application of treatments, may be delegated to allied groups by physicians. Indeed, the ascendancy of a specialty within medicine may depend on its success in delegating some aspects of work while controlling other responsibilities, such as diagnosis. Only then might those aspiring to specialty status appear as normal clinicians.

Formation of new allied occupations also depends on the capacity of other nonphysician groups to react to situations such as war. If existing allied occupations rigidly define their qualifications for membership, then they will be unable to respond to war demands for large numbers of practitioners. Moreover, commitment by these groups to paradigmatic conceptions of their work can inhibit recognition of possible opportunities, opening the way for new occupations to be created.

Once specialty groups coalesce in a given area of work, the relationships among them must be defined. According to the natural growth model, the unequal distribution of knowledge and skill between medical and allied groups would automatically determine the ordering and coordination of services in a division of labor. In this sense, physicians have an obligation, if not a legitimate right, to organize and control the work of subordinate workers possessing less expertise. It is only natural, then, that allied workers be excluded from central tasks of diagnosis and be subjected to routine supervision.

Knowledge and technique, however, may be resources used by groups of workers to justify a structure of occupational domination and subordination. To control allied workers physicians must make a successful claim to greater competence; only then can physicians argue that the rightful management of subordinate workers is their duty. Aspiring allied workers must be willing, in turn, to accept a subordinate status with little effective control over their own knowledge base and the parameters of their actual work.

For both groups the division of labor can be a mode of furthering occupational self-interest by securing markets for their services. Physicians may see the construction of a division of labor as an opportunity to control competition from allied groups by bringing them under their supervision as well as a way to enhance their own status. Allied groups may use the division of labor as a means to fight their competitors. Closer ties with medicine may be a way to gain a protective umbrella and a device to improve commodity definition. Yet what appears to be an immediate gain to allied groups may be in reality part of a long-term process of institutionalization and subordination to medicine.

Effective control over a division of labor by physicians entails more than domination of subordinate workers. Physicians also have to place themselves strategically between other medical specialties and allied occupations. To do this, closure must be achieved around a specific body of knowledge and an assortment of techniques which can justify the granting of official specialty status by the medical profession. Only then can a group of physicians claim a special and unique right to direct the work of subordinates in a division of labor that they alone dominate. Once again, the events of history may provide the opportunities to make this claim.

Yet strategies of control do not always succeed and may be frustrated by allied group opposition. Continued dependence on medicine, particularly on an individual specialty, may be seen by allied workers as an impediment to expanding demand for their services. The most effective strategy to lessen their subordination is to question the legitimacy of the division of labor itself. Allied groups may challenge the authority of a medical specialty to control their work and define the parameters of their competence on the grounds that physicians do not have exclusive and fundamental competence over a body of knowledge or set of techniques. Thus, in hospital settings allied groups may oppose administrative and professional control by a specific medical specialty. In the private, fee-for-service market, allied occupations may question their subordination to medicine in general and pursue licensing legislation allowing them to become independent practitioners. If successful with these and other expansionist tactics, the market aspirations of allied groups may lead to a redefinition of the role of the physician as more of a consultant than a manager, and to termination of a specialty's power to dominate the division of labor.

The division of labor may also become an arena for contest with other groups of physicians. This is most likely if a specialty's closure strategies fail, thus opening its domain to specialties on its boundary. Disputes may break out over the right to manage allied workers and to provide services to a discrete market of patients. The effect of such a jurisdictional battle is to question whether certain physicians have a legitimate claim to specialty status and dominance in a division of labor. Clearly, then, these local conflicts between adjacent medical specialties are as significant to the evolution of a medical division of labor as are challenges from allied workers; both may engender the demise of a specialty's occupational power.

Rehabilitation Medicine

If the significance of the market model to the problems of specialization and coordination of work could be established, policymakers would certainly be in a better position than they are now to evaluate proposals to remedy fragmentation and halt its further progress. Yet the market model is only a logical construct, and therefore requires the collection of empirical information that allows one to judge the degree to which reality conforms to the model. This work conducts such a test by examining the origin and development of a single division of labor—the field of rehabilitation medicine—from the perspective of the market interests of its workers.

Practitioners in rehabilitation medicine work with disabled and chronically ill patients to improve their functional ability. They were selected for case study for three reasons. First, specialization in rehabilitation medicine not only includes physicians in the specialty of physiatry but also allied health workers in the specialties of physical therapy and occupational therapy. This provides an opportunity to examine and compare the occupational emergence of both physician and nonphysician specialties. Moreover, these specialties have, since their inception, organized rehabilitation work in a division of labor characterized by subordination of allied health workers to physicians. Thus it is possible to study the process by which professional dominance is established in the medical division of labor.

Second, the rehabilitation field has been the subject of open conflict among specialties over both occupational boundaries and control of markets for patient care. Characteristic of the tension among occupations in this division of labor was a special Interdisciplinary Forum held to discuss the "Territorial Imperatives and the Boundaries of Professional Practice in Rehabilitation."[24] This panel, composed of physiatrists, physical therapists, and occupational therapists, as well as nurses and social workers, agreed on only one thing: they all felt a "sense of threat, attack, and hostility" in their struggle with one another over the preservation and expansion of their occupational boundaries and professional autonomy.[25] As a result of such conflict a large amount of both published and unpublished source material exists on interoccupational rivalries and the negotiation of a division of labor in this field.

Third, the development of rehabilitation medicine has been ignored by sociologists and historians alike. The few casual

histories available have been written by rehabilitation practitioners and describe the "evolution" of the field from the
perspective of the natural growth model of specialization.
Typical of these histories is one by Frank Krusen, a prominent
physiatrist. Krusen claims that during the 1930s, or the "first
decade" of physiatry, physicians with a deep concern for rehabilitation of the disabled established the field.[26] This interest
in rehabilitation continued to grow, according to Krusen, such
that official specialty status was naturally granted to physiatry
in 1947 by the AMA. This specialty was necessary, to apply
the "many new and amazing electrophysical devices and instruments" to the rehabilitation of the disabled as well as to
manage adequately the "rapid" expansion of knowledge in
this field.[27] In short, he sees the rise of physiatry as a product
of technological imperative and an outgrowth of knowledge
requirements. In addition, Krusen's history takes for granted
the authority of physiatrists over allied health workers by
seeing occupational subordination as an inevitable concomi-
tant of specialization. It is clear that this field requires a historical study that suspends natural growth assumptions and
holds the division of labor as problematic.

The approach in this case study begins by examining the
occupational emergence of physiatry, physical therapy, and
occupational therapy. Chapter 2 examines the nineteenth-century roots of physiatry in the practice of electrotherapy. Attention is focused on the way a group of physicians, marginal
to the regular medical profession, first used electrical devices,
then other physical techniques, as a basis for occupational
organization. Chapter 3 considers the influence on the development of these specialties of heightened demand for rehabilitation of soldiers wounded in World War I. It discusses
how entrance into the wartime market by this group of physicians led to increased recognition by regular medicine and,
through the delegation of some of their work, the creation of
the fields of physical and occupational therapy.

The next two chapters study the organization of a division
of labor in rehabilitation medicine. Chapter 4 analyzes the
struggle by physical and occupational therapy between the
wars to secure a place in the medical division of labor. It

describes how the relationships entered into with medicine required allied groups to sacrifice autonomy over their work. Chapter 5 looks at how physiatrists used their improved position during World War II to gain official specialty status and how physical therapists in particular were placed firmly under the control of medicine. The implications of these events are explored for the development, by midcentury, of a medically controlled division of labor in rehabilitation, with relationships and tasks defined through formal agreements and licensing laws. Finally, Chapter 6 investigates the ability of physiatrists to maintain their dominance over the rehabilitation division of labor. Attempts by allied groups to free themselves from subordination as well as moves by competing medical specialities to encroach on physiatry's domain are assessed.

2

The Bases for Specialization, 1890–1917

Throughout most of the nineteenth century the regular medical profession was hard pressed by competition from medical sects and by internal competition resulting from an "oversupply" of practitioners. The medical sects were especially critical of the "heroic" medicine predominant in the first half of the century which often relied on large doses of drugs and methods such as bloodletting for routine treatment. By contrast, regular medicine's competitors called for more benign therapies, such as fresh air, water, exercise, and diet, which for many centuries were used to treat the sick. In a medical profession oriented toward achieving dramatic results, little room existed for these seemingly simple therapies. Those both inside and outside the medical profession who championed natural agents were attacked by regular practitioners as quacks.

This competition was reduced in the latter half of the nineteenth century, bringing the medical profession closer to achieving its goal of unification. By conceiving of specialties as equal in status and as necessary for pursuit of scientific advancement, economic competition within the profession was channeled in a way that minimized the threat to unification. Justified on the basis of technological and scientific complexity, competitive economic activity was defused of its divisive potential. At the same time, the invocation of science as the basis for the organization of the profession provided a sense of shared mission cutting across all specialties. As a result of this increasing unification and as a powerful force for further unification, the medical profession obtained licensing legislation granting monopolistic powers.

With the growing power of the organized profession, specialized segments were reluctant to openly compete with or be critical of the practices of regular physicians. Instead they openly courted the regular profession as represented by the AMA, which, paradoxically, required seeking acceptance from competitors within the profession. To gain acceptance, these segments did not criticize dominant theories of disease and treatment. They associated their own scientific techniques with currently accepted theories and criticized external, lay competitors whose methods were characterized as unscientific. In addition, segments had to be cautious in claiming specialty status since this might draw attention to their potential competition with general practitioners. This ambiguous position posed strategic problems for nascent specialties. The overall result was the disappearance of diverse theories of disease and treatment typical of sectarian medicine during the nineteenth century.

As we will see, those physicians who promoted electricity as an alternative to heroic medicine laid the organizational and ideological foundations for what eventually became the modern specialty of physical medicine and rehabilitation. These electrotherapeutists organized professional associations solely around electrical devices. This served both to distinguish their modern scientific approach from that of the dissident sects and to define their commodity for market identification. The electrotherapeutic associations, however, were unable to gain the regular medical profession's acceptance of their methods and organizations. In response to this rejection they enlarged the base of their claimed expertise to include a variety of physical agents existing on the margins of conventional medicine and adopted a more aggressive posture toward internal competitors.

Electricity: A Base for Organization

Early Champions of Electricity

The modern interest in electricity as a medical cure started when William Gilbert, physician to Queen Elizabeth, published his treatise on magnetism in 1600. But not until the middle of the eighteenth century did scientists, physicians, clerics, and lay healers seriously begin to explore the medical applications of electricity. One of the first to do so was a young German physician, Christian Kratzenstein, who in 1744 found that electricity increased his pulse rate and made it easier to sleep. Within a short time he reported using electricity successfully on patients with physical paralysis and mental diseases, such as hysteria in women.[1] In colonial America, interest in the use of electricity in medicine was stimulated by Benjamin Franklin's *Experiments in Electricity*, published in 1753. While Franklin considered using electric shock to cure palsy, his experiments with paralyzed patients were disappointing. Despite his findings, Franklin thought that electricity produced some "lifting of the spirits."[2]

The popularity of electrotherapy peaked in the 1770s, particularly in France and England. Instrument makers and mechanics improved and promoted new electrical machines and wrote extensively on electrotherapy.[3] Although physicians seemed less convinced of electricity's medical benefits, machines were installed as early as 1768 in London's Middlesex Hospital and in 1777 at St. Bartholomew's.[4] These devices, however, were rarely used by the staff. By the 1790s interest in the application of electricity to medicine markedly diminished in Europe.

Interest in electrotherapy persisted somewhat longer in America. One physician, T. Gale, started using electrotherapy in his private practice in Saratoga County, New York, and was permitted to study the effects of static electricity on yellow fever patients in Bellevue Hospital in 1798.[5] In 1802 he published *Electricity or Ethereal Fire* to demystify the use of electricity so "that any man of common ingenuity may perfectly understand the benefits . . . and the effects of the electric shocks." Gale went on to describe an electrical machine "which any man may build for himself, at 2 or 3 dollars cost and little labour," and which could be used to cure as well as prevent, among other things, headaches, pleurisy, sore throats, small-pox, measles, consumption, cancer, drowning, and dysentery. More than just a polemic for medical electricity or a mechanic's manual for constructing and operating machines, Gale's book also detailed the appropriate electrical treatment for each of the various diseases covered. In cases of "fever," for example, he recommended first passing eight to ten shocks from the right hand to the left, making sure not to injure the patient, but expecting trembling and faintness to occur, and then passing twelve to fifteen shocks from the sides of the neck to the bottom of the feet, adjusting the strength of the shock according to the patient's sensation and stopping when perspiration became rapid. Two or three hours later the whole treatment was to be repeated.[6]

While works such as Gale's led to greater use of electricity by lay practitioners and patients themselves, physicians in the early part of the nineteenth century showed little interest in it. In fact, the use of medical electricity was branded as quackery by state medical societies and major medical journals. An 1844 issue of the *Boston Medical and Surgical Journal*, for example, singled out and condemned John B. Cross, a self-proclaimed "neurologist and electrician," for circulating a letter heralding the discovery of a "new remedial power of the electric current" for use on patients afflicted with an "endless list of aches, pains and diseases. . . . How modest! . . . The world is full of abominations and Boston is still the paradise of quacks."[7]

Although the regular medical profession at midcentury continued to be skeptical of and hostile to electricity, a few individual physicians started using electrotherapy as a last resource in incurable cases of "nervous affliction."[8] An even smaller number of regular physicians tried to popularize electrotherapy among their colleagues. One of them, A. C. Garratt, a Boston physician, observed the use of medical electricity in Europe and after twenty years of general practice in America became its first full-time specialist in electrotherapy.[9] He went on to write an electrotherapeutics textbook for medical students because in his opinion previous works were only argumentative and did not give "clear and precise directions as to where, when and how to employ electricity as a remedy."[10] The first chapters in his text are devoted to electrophysiology and electrical instruments. The core of the book is a detailed discussion of the applications of electricity to gynecological, surgical, nervous, and "spastic" diseases.

Another physician, George Beard, discovered while in medical school at Yale that electricity relieved his indigestion and nervousness. Beard moved to New York City in 1865 and with his close friend, Alphonse Rockwell, became partners in medical practice and spent much of their time investigating medical electricity.[11] After Beard published two papers on the subject, he wrote a book with Rockwell on electrotherapy. In its preface, they bemoaned the fact that "there are comparatively few in the profession who have given the subject sufficient heed" and that "empirics and charlatans have thus far had the field mostly to themselves." It was time, they claimed, "to wrest the medical employment of electricity from the hands of these selfish harpies."[12]

These occasional attempts at popularization had little impact on the medical profession. A review of Beard and Rockwell's book charged that the authors were overly enthusiastic and biased in their approach. "For like theology, electrotherapeutics has two distinct methods, that of faith and that of doubt, and it strikes us that what some of the old theologians taught, 'to doubt is to be damned,' must be the creed of the prominent electrotherapeutists." As an example, the reviewer cited Beard and Rockwell's claim that "pain caused by the prick of a pin is less sensitively felt when a strong faradic current is passed through the part where the puncture is made," and facetiously retorted: "Probably a redhot iron would also have an anesthetizing influence, so that a prick of a pin during its application would not seriously incommode the patient."[13] Shortly after publication of their book Rockwell asked to read a paper at the New York Medical Society, but was turned down on the grounds that electrotherapy was advocated only by quacks.

Physicians Organize

Toward the end of the nineteenth century medical electricity became somewhat more popular among regular physicians. An 1879 editorial in the first American electrotherapy journal hailed this change in the profession's attitude when only a few years earlier "those manifesting any interest in electrology were looked upon with suspicion, and if not actually branded as charlatans, were at least sneered at and avoided by the large majority of physicians."[14] Electrotherapy journals argued that this growth in popularity was due to technical advances that increased the reliability of electrical apparatus.

Electrotherapy's biggest boost came from the sudden enthusiasm of obstetricians and gynecologists for this technique. Considered by some to be a "panacea" for the treatment of women's ills, electrotherapy also allowed these physicians to distinguish themselves from other practitioners in a field plagued with an overabundance of medical men and midwives.[15] Its chief proponent was Georges Apostoli of Paris, who advocated electricity for uterine disease and tumors. By 1887 Apostoli achieved enough international recognition for the American Gynecological Society to invite him as a special guest at its twelfth annual meeting.[16]

Although many obstetricians and gynecologists refused to endorse electrotherapy, and some went as far as labeling it a "piece of rot,"[17] several American physicians, including William Harvey King, went to Paris to study under Apostoli. After graduating from the New York Homeopathic Medical College in 1882, King set up practice in New York City and taught obstetrics at his former college. He became interested in electrotherapy and sought instruction in its use, but was disappointed because no medical school taught the subject and fewer than a dozen electrotherapeutists practiced in New York City.[18] After spending a year with Apostoli, King returned to New York and began work on an electrotherapeutics textbook, published in 1889,[19] and became editor of the *Journal of Electro-Therapeutics* in 1890.

The first electrotherapy society was organized by George

Betton Massey, a Philadelphia gynecologist. In 1890 he sent letters to regular physicians known to be interested in electrotherapy suggesting the formation of a professional association. The initial organizing meeting of the American Electro-Therapeutic Association was held in January 1891 at the New York Academy of Medicine. The fourteen participants, regular physicians from New York City and Philadelphia, elected Massey the first president of the association.[20] An arrangement was made with the AMA to publish the proceedings of their meetings in the *Journal of the American Medical Association (JAMA)*.

On invitation, a small group of homeopathic physicians met at King's office in New York City on October 6, 1892, and organized a second association called the National Society of Electro-Therapeutics. Unlike the American Electro-Therapeutic Association, several of the society's twenty-seven charter members were from outside the New York-Philadelphia area, from places like Chicago, Cleveland, and the District of Columbia.[21] King became the society's first president and the *Journal of Electro-Therapeutics*, which he edited, its official organ.

Given the competitive situation between homeopaths and the regular profession, the two electrotherapeutic groups were largely independent of one another. Membership in the American Electro-Therapeutic Association was at this time open only to physicians who could also meet the membership requirements of the AMA. While the homeopathic National Society of Electro-Therapeutics allowed any physician to join it, there were no regular physicians in its ranks. Despite their common interest in electrotherapeutics, there was no cooperation between the two organizations. In 1896, for example, they both held annual meetings at the same time but in two different cities.[22]

Both groups had similar goals and pursued similar strategies. The AMA-aligned American Electro-Therapeutic Association was organized to overcome resistance to electrotherapy. At its second annual meeting, the association's president stated, "Never has a nobler agency for cure been more ignobly ignored. . . . Electrotherapy has too long been left to the designing, the ignorant and the incompetent."[23]

Members of the association were especially concerned about the problems they encountered when presenting papers to groups of regular physicians.[24] Many electrotherapeutists expressed enthusiasm about the possibility of discussing electrotherapy "without the controversial digressions that marred the reception of electrical papers in other societies."

The primary goal of the National Society of Electro-Therapeutics was to have its methods and organization accepted by the medical profession. Such recognition was important for electrotherapeutists so they could develop the commodity status of their service. Only then could the society get some guarantee of a market through referrals and assistance in restricting the practice of nonphysicians. To gain this recognition, the society and its publications were conciliatory and not sectarian. Rarely was the regular medical profession attacked, and then it was only the most heroic surgical practices that were criticized. For example, one article in their journal noted that "at last electricity . . . is superseding the knife and narcotics in the treatment of the chronic diseases of women. When you reflect that all New York is gone mad over laparotomies and hysterectomies . . . we need not be ashamed to say that we are going at least to try to cure uterine fibroma with galvinism before resorting to the knife."[25] The *Journal of Electro-Therapeutics* even published announcements and summaries of the rival American Electro-Therapeutic Association's annual meetings and articles by regular physicians who were association members. However, neither the association nor *JAMA* published any articles by members of the homeopathic group of electrotherapeutists or mentioned the society except for occasional references to the "homeopathic fungus."[26]

At this stage the goal of the society was not to establish an exclusive organization based on special expertise but to entice physicians to join the group and to use medical electricity.[27] The physician should at least look into electricity, argued the society, "for if disease can be cured more safely, surely, and speedily by electricity than by other measures, he would be remiss in his great responsibility if he did not either make use of it himself or advise its use by someone who is familiar with it!"[28] Moreover, an article in the *Journal of Electro-Thera-*

peutics entitled "Will It Pay?" suggested that physicians would find it profitable to use electricity in the treatment of disease.[29] The society was open to all physicians "interested in the development of electricity as an adjunct in therapeutics [and] it is not meant exclusively for those who devote themselves to electricity as a specialty."[30] While it was held that electrotherapy could only be performed by a physician with a thorough knowledge of pathology, no claim was made about needing specialized expertise. It was felt that the "special knowledge required of electrotherapeutics . . . is not great, and any physician of ordinary ability can master the technicalities in a few months." The necessary technical knowledge, according to King, included an understanding of how different batteries worked and how they were mechanically constructed. The physician "who is dependent entirely upon an expert electrician to repair his battery every time it needs it will make a failure in the practice of electrotherapeutics."[31]

Organizationally, the strategy of both electrotherapeutic groups was to launch a crusade to gain as many members as possible. Within one year of its founding the National Society of Electro-Therapeutics reported a membership of 100.[32] By 1893 the American Electro-Therapeutic Association had 67 members, and in 1896 an amendment to increase the membership was passed because so many candidates expressed interest in joining.[33] Three years later nearly 90 physicians were Fellows of the association.[34]

Despite this goal, persistent uncertainty remained about whether the field of electrotherapy should constitute a specialty. Two of the society's presidential addresses explicitly encouraged specialization. The 1896 address, entitled "The Electro-Therapeutist as a Specialist," was the first statement for electrotherapy as a distinct specialty. It argued that all physicians should be knowledgeable about electric treatment, but that they should send more difficult cases to specialists in this field.[35] At the 1898 meeting, the presidential address discussed the relationship of an electrotherapeutic specialty to other specialties, particularly surgery, and minimized the possibility of conflict between them. "Let the surgeon turn over to the electrotherapeutist those cases which can be treated more successfully by electricity than by the knife, and the electrotherapeutist should in return refer to the surgeon those cases which require his services."[36]

Another major concern of the society was to gain the regular profession's assistance in eliminating "quacks." Confident that the medical profession could eliminate such lay competition, the *Journal* commented: "the time is past for quackery and quack doctors to have any influence against the united efforts of the medical profession."[37] If electrotherapy were made readily available by regular physicians, consumers would choose it rather than the ministrations of quacks.[38]

Particularly upsetting to physician electrotherapeutists were electrical devices sold directly to patients by lay electrotherapeutists having no formal training. King complained that "the number of electric belts advertised is legion. Added to these are electric brushes, electric disks for wearing on a string around the neck; electric garters and electric suspensory bandages to invigorate the vitality of the male sexual organs."[39] One such device, the electric massage roller, was purported to take off weight on "women with excessive hip and waist development, and men with large abdomens," remedy sleeplessness, fatigue, cold feet, and balding, and, in combination with the electric vacuum cup, enlarge and firm up women's breasts.[40] Anyone could call himself an electrician and obtain a certificate from one of the many electrical colleges all over the country giving training in the use of these devices. The largest of these, the National College of Electro-Therapeutics in Lima, Ohio, offered a correspondence course on the subject for twenty dollars and included in the fee a copy of "The Electro-Therapeutic Guide" and a diploma awarding the degree of Master of Electro-Therapeutics (M.E.). The course provided no instruction in medicine or surgery.

The society was careful to distinguish its electrotherapy from that of nonphysician competitors and to associate its own practice with modern science. In a typical editorial King insisted that electrotherapy was not, as quacks claimed, a cure-all, and bemoaned their "exaggerated reports" of electrical cures, sarcastically remarking that "there need be no fear of anyone dying, if people would only go to them for electrical treatment."[41] The electrotherapeutists admitted that their methods did not always work. Just as regular physicians encountered failure in their practices, "disease does not always yield at once to medicines, and why should we expect more of electricity?"[42] Moreover, electrical treatment might fail, they claimed, because "nearly every physician has a battery that he uses upon occasion; but in how many instances is that same battery out of order, or of the family battery type—an obsolete instrument."[43] Or such treatment might fail because the physician simply lacked basic knowledge of electrotherapeutics, as the following anecdote suggested:

> How much does the average physician know of electro-therapeutics when he receives his diploma? The majority of them know absolutely nothing of this branch. A friend of mine . . . was called upon to treat by electricity a patient suffering from neuralgia of the face and scalp. The office outfit consisted of the old-fashioned bluestone battery. The patient was a man weighing 180 pounds; he was given a sponge electrode in each hand and told to place them upon his temples while the physician turned on the current. Not having a milliamperemeter or a rheostat, the whole force of the battery was turned on at once; the patient fell to the floor like a lump of lead. When the physician and patient recovered from the shock, they both concluded they would try some other method of cure, the patient declaring that he had no further use for electricity; and the physician immediately after commenced the study of electrotherapeutics.[44]

The "average physician," according to the society, did not appreciate that electrotherapy was fast becoming an "exact science having clearly marked indications for application to different diseases" much as did medical science.[45] One electrotherapeutic physician highlighted the legitimating power of science by declaring that "the statements in our papers and discussions of results obtained carry but little weight unless there is a rational explanation of methods adopted, showing the appearance of scientific research."[46] In addition, electrotherapeutists claimed their field had a "scientific foundation" based on knowledge about the properties of electricity itself and its effects on physiology, as well as the mechanics of electrical apparatus. Thus, one writer sought to distinguish the therapeutic effects of electricity from other physical measures. While admitting that "some of the results in electrotherapeutics are due in a measure, although not in great measure . . . to physical effects," he went on to emphasize the chemical actions precipitated by electrical stimulation. He pointed to the modification of physiological functions whereby some were increased (e.g., salivary secretion) and some decreased (e.g., urine). Electricity was described as a "tonic of a very high order" which produces the "requisite degree of tension of the nervous system." Belying the existing scientific understanding of electrotherapy, he stated that "the numerous branch currents, going to and fro, act as so many shuttlecocks, keeping every atom in incessant disturbance" and electricity should be used whenever "a constitutional tonic influence is called for."[47]

Enlarging the Base

Internal Competition

The attempt in the 1890s to change the attitude of regular physicians toward electrotherapy achieved mixed results. On the one hand, the electrotherapeutists gained some acceptance for their methods from individual physicians and hospitals. While practitioners publicly criticized electrotherapy, many used it in their private offices. Estimates are that by the early 1900s some 25,000 physicians at least owned an electric battery and half this number routinely used electrotherapy as one of their treatments.[48] Even some hospitals, such as Massachusetts General Hospital in Boston, had faculty positions in electrotherapeutics and a few medical schools offered instruction on the subject.[49]

On the other hand, electrotherapy was still considered a marginal medical practice, and most regular physicians were unwilling to give it any formal recognition. Harsh denouncements of electrotherapeutics continued to appear in the major medical journals. As one physician observed, "the very term 'electric specialist' stinks to heaven . . . a large element of these lightning-jerkers, let us call them, are the most monumental charlatans that one could well find. And of all the charlatans I ever met, the electric gentlemen is the cleverest— A, No. 1, gilt-edged."[50] Going on to explain why electrotherapy was so commonly used by physicians, this author noted that medicine was steadily growing more difficult for the general practitioner because there was "no longer enough acute disease to go around" with the result that "many have taken up the electric battery in self-defense. And as electric treatments happen to be all the fashion at present, they are working the lead for all it is worth, their zeal being, if anything, surpassed by that of the serene dodos who troop to their offices . . . always looking for improvement, which somehow or other doesn't materialize."[51] Comprehensive annual reviews of medical progress such as the *American Yearbook of Medicine and Surgery* typically devoted less than two pages each year to medical electricity and then only to acknowledge its possible use in cases of chronic pain or psychological disorders.

When the association absorbed the *Journal of Electro-Therapeutics* in 1902, electrotherapeutists began to deemphasize electrotherapy and incorporate other therapies as their base. Now called the *Journal of Advanced Therapeutics*, it became the official organ of the American Electro-Therapeutic Association. The new editor, William B. Snow, was a leading member of the association. After graduating from Columbia's College of Physicians and Surgeons in 1885, Snow started to research the effects of static electricity on infections. He joined the association in 1899 and became its president four years later. Referred to as "the dean of physical therapy," Snow was its chief advocate for nearly thirty years until his early radiological experiments led to his death as an "x-ray martyr."[52] Snow and the editors that followed him never mentioned the National Society of Electro-Therapeutics and only one reference was made to King, the previous editor, noting that he held the chair in physical therapeutics at the New York Homeopathic Medical School.[53] Clearly, the association did not want any connection with homeopathy. Still criticized by the medical profession, homeopathy was in a general decline.

The *Journal of Advanced Therapeutics* no longer restricted itself to electrical devices, as had the earlier journal. Its fifteen departments included thermotherapy, hydrotherapy, psychotherapy, phototherapy, mechanical vibration therapy, climatology, exercise, and dietetics. This group of diverse therapies constituted a grab bag of practices unpopular with the regular medical profession and was eventually trimmed down to those easily linked by the concept of externally applied physical agents such as heat, water, massage, and electricity. The editor coined the term "physical therapeutics" for their work and linked these centuries-old therapies for the first time.[54] "With the development of rational medicine the physician learns more and more to appreciate the natural forces essential to life, light, heat, water and other chemical constituents of the body." The physician, therefore, should use "the energizing forces of nature—light, heat, and electricity."[55] The "natural" treatment for "neurasthenia" or depression, for example, involved all or most of the following treatments: a quick jet douche on the spine, a carbonic acid bath for twenty minutes, gymnastics, abdominal massage and vibration, cold applications to the precordial region, diuretic drinks and calomel mixed with bicarbonate of soda, electrostatic baths, electric douches, and faradization.[56]

While the *Journal's* new editors did broaden its scope, the major emphasis until World War I continued to be on electrical treatments. Other therapies were considered secondary. In fact, some members expressed concern that too much attention would be given to "borderland studies" such as x-ray, light, or mechanical vibration, and not enough to the "electrical modalities proper."[57] And an attempt in 1906 to change the name of the association to reflect the inclusion of other physical measures was rejected; it was felt that electricity was included in these other measures as a "means of power or as a source of the other physical measures."[58]

Clearly, these diverse therapies had no inherent connection except that all were medical practices existing on medicine's periphery. They were combined because a group of practitioners were unsuccessful in their attempt to organize around the technology of electricity. To gain recognition the electrotherapeutists developed a broader base to launch further claims for the general utility of their measures.[59] While the association remained concerned primarily with gaining the profession's acceptance of electricity, they now had a basis for claiming the use of therapies dependent on "natural" forces and for restricting their use to practitioners who understood the scientific principles underlying them.

This process of incorporating other therapies began when the electrotherapeutists staked a claim to the recently discovered x-ray. Characterized by King as one of the "great possibilities of electricity," the electrotherapeutists were especially quick to recognize the x-ray's potential usefulness.[60] The electrotherapeutists displayed immediate interest in x-rays, reprinting Wilhelm Roentgen's original paper in their journal early in 1896. By 1898 over forty articles appeared in the *Journal* on "this mighty diagnostic and remedial agent" ranging from discussions of its value in locating bullets in wounded soldiers and coins stuck in children's throats to its value in removing freckles and facial hair.

Other physicians, however, became solely interested in the x-ray itself and developed a journal and association prior to the turn of the century. At first they denied the need for special knowledge or skill to use the x-ray and promoted its general adoption by physicians. This strategy was similar to that used by the electrotherapeutists. As one x-ray proponent wrote: "Is the art of manipulating a superb Crooke's tube difficult and does it take long experience? On the contrary it is simplicity itself and full instruction in the best technique involves but a couple of hours time . . . x-rays are available for the general profession. Their use need not be confined to a few."[61] But as lay competition increased, these physicians called for an exclusive, specialized practice. One author suggested that nonphysicians were mainly concerned with financial gain and that they would cause a decline in radiography. Seeking to develop "Roentgenogram ethics," he declared that radiography should be practiced only by physicians.[62] The argument for exclusive, specialized practice was not based on claimed medical expertise in interpreting x-rays. Rather, technical complexity and economic competition, thinly veiled behind concerns over ethics, were the bases on which some argued for specialization.[63]

At first the National Society of Electro-Therapeutics did not see any grounds for conflict with this potential rival. The beginning of the *X-Ray Journal* in 1897 and the first meeting of the Roentgen Ray Society of America in 1900 were announced in the *Journal of Electro-Therapeutics,* and "best wishes" were extended to the new enterprises.[64] Although the electrotherapeutists saw the x-ray as naturally falling within the confines of electrical treatment, they did not try to establish an exclusive claim over its use. Their principal goal still was to gain acceptance of electrotherapy and to promote the use of electrical devices for all types of diseases regardless of specialty.

Although electrotherapeutists originally organized around the use of electricity for gynecological conditions, they felt that the use of electrical devices should not be limited to any specialty, and that no specialty was complete without them.[65] This conceptualization was one reason for their own ambiguity about what their structural relationship should be within the profession. For example, some felt that it was not possible to develop a specialty based on a single agent like electricity, and therefore the focus should continue to be on this therapy's value for the whole profession.[66] In this regard electrotherapeutists posed little threat to more narrowly based specialties.

This posture changed to a more imperialistic one when the *Journal* was taken over by the American Electro-Therapeutic Association. There are several possible reasons for this new, politically aggressive stance. First, it may have been that the association's connection to regular medicine made it feel more secure in launching direct attacks at current medical practices and the resistance to electrical means of therapy. Second, it may have been the association's aggressive posture that resulted in its ascendance and the society's decline. Finally, the lack of real progress in convincing the profession of the value of their techniques, in addition to the increased internal competition, may have resulted in the escalation of their tactics.

Now viewed as a competitor, radiology came under attack.

The electrotherapeutists claimed that as specialists in electricity, they were the most competent physicians to use this technique: "no body of physicians are so well qualified to consider the scientific employment of the x-ray in medical practice as those who have devoted years to the study of electrotherapeutics."[67] Although they were silent about what constituted their special qualifications and scientific understanding, variously referring to x-rays as "photography of the invisible," "electrical vision," and the result of "ether vibrations,"[68] they were vocal when it came to stressing the "timidity" of radiologists who only used x-rays for diagnostic purposes.

Even though the *Journal* frequently published articles on the therapeutic value of x-rays, a small group of electrotherapeutists tried to take over one of the radiologists' own journals so that they could espouse their conception of the x-ray to a wider audience. In 1902 a number of electrotherapeutists who belonged to the Roentgen Society successfully gained control of the *American X-Ray Journal*, a private venture published by Dr. Heber Robarts of St. Louis. A radiologist's later historical account described their struggle: "a fringe of electrotherapists attempted to either control or sabotage this poorly organized society, much to the embarrassment of Dr. Robarts. They attempted to euchre the editor out of his journal and finally succeeded."[69]

There were also increased attacks on the other internal competitors, surgeons and neurologists. The electrotherapeutists called for a "halt in this lust for operative surgery" and the replacement of surgical procedures with safer and more effective physical therapies such as electricity, hot air, and water.[70] Particularly in cases of malignant disease, surgeons were accused of mutilating patients without curing them and of ignoring the therapeutic benefits of the x-ray, which the electrotherapeutist could provide.[71] Since some surgeons were starting to use the x-ray as a therapy, this too was criticized by the electrotherapeutists, again on the basis of special knowledge and skill that they, not surgeons, possessed. "It would be as reasonable for a physician who had acquired no skill in surgery to attempt to perform a laparotomy as for a surgeon who did not know a volt from an ampere, or a high tube from a low one, to employ the x-ray in the treatment of cancer."[72]

Neurologists were attacked for relying on psychotherapy.[73] This attack was ironic because psychotherapy was for a brief period considered by electrotherapeutists to be a "department" of physical therapeutics. The electrotherapeutists' interest in psychotherapy proved short-lived, however. It turned to antagonism when critics suggested that electrotherapy's main value lay in the psychological reaction of the patient to electrical devices.[74] By only using "suggestion," the electrotherapeutists claimed that neurologists were not treating the underlying physical causes of nervous disease which had to be eliminated to effect a cure. While neurologic techniques failed to get at these underlying causes, it was argued, physical therapeutics could succeed.[75]

As a complement to these attacks, the electrotherapeutists tried to secure a formal position within the regular profession by creating a "Committee on Affiliation with the AMA," but this effort was subsequently rebuffed by the AMA. The association then called for a section on physical therapeutics in the AMA to establish the legitimacy of their methods.[76] These sections were generally the first step in the granting of formal AMA recognition to segments within the profession. However, this request was rejected in 1905.[77] Formal recognition was again denied in 1907 when the electrotherapeutists petitioned the AMA to institute a physical therapeutics section and called on it to follow the precedent set by the British Medical Association, the British Academy of Medicine, and the New York Academy of Medicine, each of which had recently created a section on electrotherapeutics.[78] The Association continued to pursue this goal unsuccessfully over the next several years.

External Competition

The incorporation of other physical therapies by the electrotherapeutists also led to conflict with nonphysicians. One proponent of "manual therapy" held that "the electrotherapeutist deals especially with physical methods of treatment, so that manual therapy falls naturally within his province."

Such therapy was not to be left to the "indiscriminating masseur, nor the superficial frictions and kneadings of the nurse," but rather "must be applied by a trained physician who possesses the surgeon's knowledge of anatomy, the physiologist's knowledge of function, and a knowledge of abnormal structure and altered function." The author noted regretfully that physicians usually turn over such treatment to the masseur or nurse "whose interest in the case frequently centers on the fee at the end of the task." Because of this practice "hundreds of laymen . . . have received a smattering of electrotherapeutical methods while acting as assistants in the office of the honest and legitimate physician, and have gone forth to prostitute the system by resorting to the nefarious schemes of quackery."[79]

The fact that many states legally recognized these non-physician practitioners greatly concerned the electrotherapeutists.[80] In New Jersey, for example, the law regulating the practice of medicine and surgery allowed anyone to treat patients with electrotherapy if they had seven years experience with it and graduated from an electrotherapeutic school.[81] Of special concern were osteopaths and masseurs who sought state legislation protecting the same physical techniques claimed by electrotherapeutists as part of medicine. In reaction to this threat, the editor of the *Journal of Advanced Therapeutics* urged national adoption of a New York Court of Records decision that defined medical practice as the use of any means by a "person holding himself or herself out as able to cure diseases, with a view to relieve, heal, or cure, and having for its object the prevention, healing, remedying, cure, or alleviation of disease." It was suggested that the American Electro-Therapeutic Association appoint a committee to press for such legislation so that the public would be protected.[82]

In sum, the increasing importance of licensure pushed the electrotherapeutists to secure legal protection for their practice. During a period when the medical profession was gaining a legal monopoly over most types of medical practice, its boundaries would be determined by battles at the profession's "periphery" among specialty segments claiming areas of practice considered outside regular medicine by most physicians. In the process, opposition by these segments to irregulars and quacks led to the elimination or restriction of their practice and to the formal incorporation of segments into the profession. By guarding and extending medicine's perimeters, the electrotherapeutic segment prevented an ambivalent medical profession from closing the door on it.

The Response to AMA Rejection

Between 1910 and 1917 the position of the association and electrotherapeutics in general did not improve markedly and even declined in certain respects. Frustrated that more individual physicians were not interested in using electrotherapy or in joining the association, the electrotherapeutists felt that they were becoming increasingly isolated and ignored. Fears of "stagnation" were expressed by association officers as membership leveled off at slightly over two hundred and as "so many static machines are idle in the offices of physicians."[83] In his 1913 presidential address, Francis Howard Humphris was moved to remark: "I fear that it cannot be denied . . . we are like St. John the Baptist—'the voice of one crying in the wilderness.'"[84] After Humphris's inauguration, *JAMA* published even fewer articles on electrotherapeutics.

Failure to gain recognition led to increased impatience by the electrotherapeutists. Some association members blamed themselves for not providing sufficient scientific proof of their methods and for making excessive claims about electrotherapy's potential to cure.[85] Others blamed the medical profession for its ignorance and bitterly decried the accusation of quackery directed at them by regular physicians. One angry electrotherapeutist called for an end to ridicule leveled at his colleagues "when they mention their [physical techniques] value or importance in medical meetings by those who know little or nothing of their indications or use" and who "discredit them in the community as they would a quack or osteopath."[86] Medical schools were criticized for not giving any instruction in their methods and for "looking dubiously upon electrotherapeutics" when instruction was given.[87] *JAMA* was even attacked for quoting people who were not well known in the field of electrotherapeutics and for using book reviewers who knew nothing about the subject.[88]

Limited recognition did come shortly thereafter when the AMA recommended medical school instruction in the "non-pharmaceutical" areas of diet, hygiene, massage, exercise, electricity, x-rays, phototherapy, thermotherapy, balneology, climatology, and psychotherapy. Following this "step in the right direction," the electrotherapeutists again pressed for recognition as a section within the AMA,[89] but again no special status was given. Although the AMA recommendation indicated that it did not want to lose these diverse therapies to irregular practitioners, neither did it want to give any special status to electrotherapy, including it instead as one among many such therapies. Thus while some recognition was given to these therapies, the association failed to have electricity singled out as extremely noteworthy.

In response to the AMA's decision, the association made some changes, including the symbolic renaming of its journal in 1916 to the *American Journal of Electrotherapeutics and Radiology*.[90] The new name was part of a larger attempt to reemphasize the centrality of electricity, despite declining interest in this sort of treatment, and to recapture the x-ray, motivated by the increased general interest in it and by the growth of organizations of radiologists who wanted to create their own specialty. Rivalry between the electrotherapeutists and radiologists led to attacks in this journal on the "exclusiveness" of those using x-rays.[91] Reversing their earlier position that it was necessary for a specialist to use x-rays, the electrotherapeutists now held that techniques could be taught to the internist. "Time was when the practice of this diagnostic art was entirely in the hands of the Roentgen specialist. But, through the labors of these workers the methods and the principles have been so elucidated that the torch may now be passed to the internist for the illumination of the devious and dark paths of clinical diagnosis."[92] The *Journal* also charged that radiologists were "unscientific monotherapists" destined to fail in their efforts because they only used a single type of treatment in their practice.[93]

This attack was part of a new strategy of condemning medical specialism and courting the favor of the general practitioner. One editorial claimed that snobbishness, exclusiveness, and resistance to innovation were typical of specialists who "like the reactionaries in politics . . . dominate the field and shut out the introduction of things which they themselves do not want recognized, and which may reflect upon their own standing."[94] Surgery, neurology, and orthopedics were singled out because they failed to adopt electrical therapies. The attack on surgery in particular was escalated to a new level through the characterization of surgeons as the "businessmen of the profession who want to control medical affairs." The imputed overreliance on surgery was directly connected to its profitability, and surgeons' resistance to physical modes of therapy was attributed to fear of losing income.[95] By contrast, general practitioners who controlled the AMA and represented a crucial source of referrals for the electrotherapeutists were lauded for being open-minded and "well disposed to progressive medicine."[96]

In siding with the recently strengthened AMA and its opposition to specialism the electrotherapeutists renounced any claim to constituting a specialty. They argued that their physical methods constituted a third branch of medicine that could serve as a complement to or a substitute for pharmaceutical and surgical treatment. By emphasizing their ability to treat a wide variety of acute medical problems, the electrotherapeutists linked themselves to the traditional model of medical practice. In a medical market based on the acute problems of a paying clientele, there was little alternative except to adapt to the existing model.

When the United States first became involved in World War I, organized electrotherapeutists had a mixed record of successes and failures. The initial basis for organization was the technology of electricity, but this did not constitute an inexorable force of technical innovation; technology offered an "opportunity point" for practitioners to pursue their interests. They linked this innovation to preexisting "natural" therapies to claim an organized group which represented scientific progress. The claim was more readily propagated by emphasizing a new technology than by extolling the older therapies and concepts.

Further development of the field and the alteration of its

boundaries depended on a variety of social and political processes. During this period the medical profession obtained exclusionary powers in the form of licensure. To incorporate and unite all aspects of medical treatment which could be connected to modern science, the profession adopted a more flexible posture toward practices claiming a basis in new knowledge or technology. Determining which new practice would be included within the profession's changing boundaries depended not only on the degree of scientific validation which proponents of particular therapies could claim but also on the existence of organizational structures to pursue the political and strategic activity prerequisite to acceptance by the regular medical profession.

The electrotherapeutists set their initial boundaries around a modern technology and developed organizational mechanisms in a journal and annual conferences. To establish social unity through a common language they created a committee to standardize electrical nomenclature. In pursuit of scientific legitimation they established a number of scientific committees which provided the main focus for their early activity. They also attempted to gain some control over manufacturers of electrical devices by creating a Committee to Evaluate and Standardize Apparatus. Finally, the 1915 creation of a Committee on Publicity indicates awareness of the role to be played by ideology in gaining acceptance from the profession, and in the struggle against internal and external competitors.

For the most part, however, the electrotherapeutists' desire to gain acceptance for their methods had not been fulfilled. The regular profession's reaction, as reflected in *JAMA*, typically was to call for "scientific caution" in the use of these therapies. Yet these statements did not usually resort to the harsh rhetoric directed in the past at those who espoused divergent notions of treatment.

More significant for the future was the extension of the field's original boundaries to include the diverse group of therapies then existing at the medical profession's periphery. With the decline of interest in electrical devices and the loss of the x-ray to organized radiologists, these "physical therapies" became the core of the field.

3

War and the Organization of Work, 1917–1920

Before World War I disability was not considered a medical or a social problem in America. The new "scientific" medical profession had extended its domain within the constraints provided by the fee-for-service market. Disabled people, who were generally unable to pay for lengthy professionalized care, were thus excluded from the services of the new medicine.

A new creed of social responsibility was developing, however, in a period of increasing consciousness of social problems, especially those caused by industrialization. Social reformers in the progressive era recognized and confronted for the first time the growing number of people disabled in industrial accidents. Estimates that 14,000 workers were permanently disabled every year and that over 500,000 people of working age suffered from some vocational handicap led these reformers to create organizations such as the Federation of Associations for Cripples to make known the problem and their proposed solutions. Neither was this problem lost on the medical profession during these decades of reform. Alexander Lambert, president of the AMA, responded by calling for the "salvaging" of America's industrial cripples.[1] The public sector responded as well. Several states passed workmen's compensation laws providing medical services and financial aid for the disabled.[2] The view that disability required public and private support was gaining acceptance.

World War I transformed the steady flow of industrial victims to a torrent of maimed and disabled. By May 1919, approximately 123,000 disabled soldiers returned to the United States from the American Expeditionary Forces. Following the lead of European nations, the country was forced to develop medical and rehabilitative services for soldiers wounded and disabled in the war. Medical and nonmedical organizations with an interest in this work sought to define the services offered by, and the boundaries between, different groups providing this care. The European experience, as portrayed in the words of one participant, was to be prophetic: "The man himself appears to have little voice in deciding his own future, while a battle royal between the doctor and the technical expert often rages over his mutilated body."[3]

In this chapter we will describe the conflict over the control of rehabilitation of the war wounded which occurred within the army's newly created Division of Physical Reconstruction and between it and the civilian Federal Board for Vocational Education. The latter conflict created a rigid line of demarcation between the medical and vocational aspects of rehabilitation. This division made development of comprehensive services problematic after the war. The struggles within the military medical department were critical (as was true again in World War II) for the place of physiotherapy and rehabilitation in the medical division of labor.

The War Wounded and Occupational Conflict

Internal Competition

When war broke out in Europe, the electrotherapeutists (now calling themselves physiotherapists) were still preoccupied with proving the utility of their specialty for acute care, and rejected the suggestion that their methods were most suited to chronic conditions. The specialists who were more experienced in dealing with injuries and disability were industrial physicians and orthopedic surgeons. In the early 1900s companies started to hire industrial physicians to provide immediate surgical care for accident victims. Viewed "with more or less contempt by the majority of the profession" and paid less relative to most other specialists, industrial physicians were given a boost by the passage of workmen's compensation laws just prior to the war.[4] They saw in the war an opportunity to move beyond care of the injured to prevention and protection of health, and thus to establish a more secure basis for a specialty. In 1918 a resolution to recognize industrial medicine as a specialty passed the AMA House of Delegates.[5] Industrial physicians also staked a claim to the possession of special skills that would be needed to place disabled men in civilian jobs. As one "company surgeon" argued, "the industrial physician, by the nature of his calling, will be the wisest guide in their placement in industry and in the maintenance of their productive ability."[6]

By contrast, orthopedic surgeons had a much longer history of caring for the disabled. Surgery in orthopedic cases dates to the eighteenth and early nineteenth centuries. The use of straps and braces to correct skeletal deformities also had a lengthy history. During the last half of the nineteenth century, surgical and mechanical modalities were combined to form the basis for a new specialty of orthopedic surgery. The American Orthopedic Association (AOA), formed in 1887, sought to bring together physicians using surgical and/or mechanical procedures to treat deformities and joint problems.[7] The early orthopedists were concerned about establishing a legitimate base within the profession and defining their services' uniqueness as a distinctive commodity. Externally, they emphasized their surgical skills to distinguish their work from that of competitors, such as homeopaths, chiropodists, and instrument makers.[8] Within the profession, their distinctive feature was the incorporation of simple mechanical devices, which posed problems for achieving a legitimate status as a specialty. They had to overcome a reputation as being merely a "society of buckle-and-strap men" whose claim to unique expertise was based on "a manual dexterity with tools."[9] Despite these problems, orthopedic surgeons gained official recognition in 1912 as a section in the AMA.

In May 1916, with United States involvement in the war imminent, the AOA formed a committee to represent their interests in the expanding military market. Joel Goldthwait, a graduate of Harvard Medical School and chief of orthopedics at Massachusetts General Hospital, was appointed chairman of this committee. His chief duty was to estimate the manpower and equipment needed by orthopedic hospitals should the United States enter the war. To help him make this appraisal, Goldthwait was dispatched to England in the spring of 1917 to observe the orthopedic work of the British.[10]

In July 1917 the AOA officially offered the services of its members to the surgeon general. He responded favorably to this offer and asked the AOA to prepare a guide for orthopedic practice in military camps and to place a member of its war-preparedness committee in his office.[11] One month later an advisory council was formed combining members of the AMA orthopedic surgery section and past AOA presidents to assist the surgeon general in planning for orthopedic work on a large scale. The council immediately sent letters to all orthopedic surgeons to obtain data on their qualifications and availability for service and called for expansion of training programs in orthopedic surgery to meet increased demand for such care.

Shortly thereafter, in August 1917, the surgeon general created a Division of Orthopedic Surgery in the Medical Department of the Army. Another Harvard-trained orthopedist working at Massachusetts General Hospital, Elliott Brackett, was put in charge of this division. Brackett was given a mandate by the surgeon general to provide a large number of orthopedic surgeons for service in Europe and America, to arrange for orthopedic equipment overseas, and to develop plans for orthopedic reconstruction in the United States.[12]

Creation of a separate Division of Orthopedic Surgery, however, was contrary to the desires of general surgeons. One general surgeon later argued that the need for "fundamental coordination with the mother subjects" was not fully recognized when orthopedic and head surgery were given independent status in the Medical Department of the Army. General surgery, it was felt, was no longer "a team, with suitable players, in the various fields, but a league of teams essentially competitive . . . and that this rivalry, while quite friendly, had a disorganizing tendency."[13] The general surgeons tried to regain organizational control over the orthopedic and head surgeons, but this was not accomplished until fall 1918. With the reorganization of the surgeon general's office, the Orthopedic and Head Surgery divisions became sections of the Division of General Surgery.

The surgeon general created the Division of Orthopedic Surgery for several reasons. Orthopedic surgeons had more experience working with injuries and deformities than other medical practitioners, and they used physiotherapeutic methods. Founded in 1904, the orthopedic surgeon-directed medicomechanical department of Massachusetts General Hospital was one of the first to employ massage, exercise, and hydrotherapy in a hospital. From 1908 to 1914, this department treated almost 5,000 patients with fractures, dislocations, stiff joints, deformities, sprains, arthritis, and paralysis.[14] Orthopedic surgeons like Goldthwait and Brackett, who were associated with the medicomechanical department at Massachusetts General Hospital, demonstrated their specialty's interest in caring for the crippled and deformed.[15] In 1895 Goldthwait organized the first clinic in America for adult cripples and several years later started the orthopedic ward and outpatient clinic at Massachusetts General Hospital.[16] Deeply committed to the movement among orthopedic surgeons for special education and vocational training for crippled children, Brackett helped found in 1893 the Industrial School for Crippled and Deformed Children.[17]

Realizing that this reorganization and opportunity for expansion might constitute an "epoch in the history of the specialty," orthopedic surgeons moved quickly.[18] Goldthwait's committee estimated that seventy-five to eighty percent of the expected 100,000 war wounded would need orthopedic surgery, making it necessary to create a "national orthopedic reserve." Orthopedists in this reserve, argued Goldthwait, would serve "on the front," where as assistants to general surgeons they would do acute emergency work, and in special orthopedic hospitals in America and England, where they would do reconstructive work with internists, radiologists, and anesthesiologists serving as consultants.[19] To operationalize this plan, Brackett, as head of the surgeon general's orthopedic division, immediately called for 35,000 orthopedic beds in France and 500 orthopedic surgeons to care for American soldiers who would be wounded in Europe.[20] By July 1918 over 600 orthopedic surgeons entered the military and every training camp, base hospital, and fort had at least one orthopedic officer.[21]

Orthopedic surgeons stressed the need to go beyond surgery and widen the conception of their work to include health education and vocational rehabilitation, and asserted that these military programs should be provided to the civilian population.[22] Goldthwait claimed that special exercises and proper use of the body had to be taught to recruits to make them physically fit and to the wounded to restore them for duty. It should be the orthopedic surgeon's responsibility, according to Goldthwait, to teach soldiers such things as foot exercises so that troops could hike farther and proper military posture so that weak backs could be strengthened.[23] Orthopedic surgeons also questioned, on humanitarian and economic grounds, the "old idea" of discharging a disabled soldier to civilian life without being occupationally "reconstructed."[24] Only then could war cripples "become happy, productive, wage-earning citizens, instead of boastful, consuming, idle derelicts."[25] More specifically, orthopedic surgeons maintained that their expertise should be used to determine the disabled soldier's medical and mental limitations for his previous occupation and to suggest specific training to overcome these limitations.[26] These recommendations for a new conception of orthopedic surgery, claimed Goldthwait, "should cover conditions as they exist in times of peace as well as time of war," and should be especially applicable to "that great body often spoken of as the industrial army."[27] The "great war," remarked one member of the Orthopedic Advisory

Council, was necessary to arouse orthopedic surgeons to a sense of their responsibility for the "purely civil cripple" who for so long had been ignored.[28]

For the most part, however, these plans were checked. After a series of meetings in August 1917, the surgeon general created the Division of Special Hospitals and Physical Reconstruction to handle the problems of the war wounded. The division's initial program was elaborate, embracing plans for the development of physical reconstruction hospitals, the clinical treatment and vocational training of wounded soldiers, and their placement in suitable occupations after discharge.[29] The makeup of the division indicated that other physicians desired a piece of this new reconstruction work and sought appointments in such special hospitals. General surgeons, for example, questioned Brackett and Goldthwait's plan for surgeons to care only for acute emergencies in base hospitals and orthopedists to handle restoration of maimed soldiers in special hospitals. One general surgeon remarked "there will be very little left for general surgeons to do, mostly digging out junk and bullets and sewing up wounds. The only solution is to make them [base hospitals] special hospitals."[30] General surgeons claimed they were as competent as orthopedists in caring for fractures and deformities, and therefore "should have a chance at some of these cases."[31]

Rather than being controlled by orthopedics, then, the Division of Special Hospitals and Physical Reconstruction had medical officers to represent general surgery, orthopedic surgery, head surgery, and neuropsychiatry.[32] Thus pressure from other specialists, and the limited number and skills of orthopedic surgeons, resulted in their incorporation and in the kind of broad program initially suggested by orthopedic surgeons. The internal struggle over definition and control of this new area, as well as the external struggle with civilian agencies, caused the program to remain largely inoperative for almost a year.

The orthopedic surgeons benefited by gaining an administrative status separate from general surgery. This allowed them to set up courses in civilian universities to train more orthopedic surgeons.[33] By the summer of 1918 almost 700 officers passed through special orthopedic courses offered in seven cities. Orthopedists were also assigned the task of supervising the construction of artificial limbs. This was an important step in achieving control over limb and instrument makers, a matter of concern to orthopedic surgeons for many years.[34] Another responsibility given to orthopedic surgeons was instruction in the examination and care of soldiers' feet and shoes. They were asked to provide courses on this topic to medical personnel and to write a manual on foot care and the treatment of foot ailments.[35]

In addition, orthopedic surgeons were the first to train what were later called "reconstruction aides." They sought to create a large corps of "specially trained masseurs" who could treat joint and muscle conditions, and to organize these workers into some official position.[36] These assistants had been used by orthopedic surgeons at the medicomechanical department of Massachusetts General Hospital before the war, and the department's chief assistant helped develop standards and training programs for them. Acceptance of the right of orthopedic surgeons to direct the aides was reflected in the surgeon general's requirement that applicants for these positions furnish a letter of recommendation from an orthopedic surgeon.[37] However, the authority of orthopedic surgeons to control the aides was challenged by physiotherapists. By May 1918 the aides were transferred to the recently renamed Division of Physical Reconstruction, further restricting the orthopedic surgeons' initial claims.[38]

This transfer had important consequences for organized physiotherapists. While they did not react quickly to wartime opportunities, the physiotherapists formed a war-preparedness committee in 1917 to press for use of their methods.[39] With the establishment of a physiotherapy section in the Division of Special Hospitals and Physical Reconstruction, the physiotherapists felt their methods would be represented in the war effort. Dr. Frank Granger, an instructor in physical therapeutics at Harvard and Tufts College and president of the newly renamed American Association of Electro-Therapeutics and Radiology, became director of the physiotherapy section in November 1917.[40]

It was unclear, however, who had ultimate authority over this work. Organizational charts showed that both the Division of Orthopedic Surgery and the Division of Special Hospitals and Physical Reconstruction would share authority over Orthopedic Service Reconstruction Hospitals.[41] The physiotherapists argued that the physiotherapy section should serve an advisory function and should not be controlled by medical or surgical interests since they had "in the past been hampered in not being permitted to carry out their work except under the direction of those who knew nothing of the methods or their value."[42] Despite the appointment of Granger to head the physiotherapy section, the ambiguous position of this section and the reconstruction aides would not be clarified until the external conflict between the Medical Department of the Army and other agencies interested in care of the war wounded was resolved.

External Conflict

The attempt by the Medical Department of the Army, with AMA support, to extend the medical profession's boundaries to include vocational training and placement was resisted by the Federal Board for Vocational Education and by several private agencies. The Federal Board had been formed in 1917, and not only provided an organizational base to combat the interests of the military Medical Department but also created an important precedent for federal involvement in issues relating to social welfare. The occupational interests here were not as well defined as those of the medical profession in the Medical Department of the Army, although vocational educators sought to control programs for training and placing the injured or disabled. In addition, a number of agencies established before the war, for example, the Red Cross Institute for the Crippled and Disabled, opposed the military Medical Department. These organizations brought together groups of workers who would eventually develop specific occupational identities in areas such as social work and vocational rehabilitation counseling.

The seeds for conflict were sown when the surgeon general adopted the orthopedic surgeons' plan to create a system of orthopedic reconstruction hospitals having vocational workshops and employment bureaus.[43] He announced the plan to construct nineteen of these hospitals in September 1917.[44] Lacking any legislative mandate for this decision, the surgeon general cited the War Risk Insurance Act, which promised rehabilitation of the wounded but did not specify who would do the work or make any commitment of funds.[45] The surgeon general tried to supply necessary manpower by commissioning vocational education experts as "sanitary officers" in the Medical Department of the Army, and sought to pay for the plan with Medical Department money.

The Federal Board for Vocational Education began its own study of vocational rehabilitation in August 1917 which was published as a Senate Document through a resolution introduced by "friends" of the board in the Senate.[46] The Federal Board argued for public status and administration of the program, and opposed military discipline of injured men except during the stage of physical cure.[47] It also claimed that the War Risk Insurance Act did not provide the surgeon general with authority to proceed with his plans, and recommended that program control be under an existing agency experienced in the administration of vocational training.[48] In addition, they submitted a detailed plan of services to be provided and who would be responsible for them. The plan called for placing civilian vocational experts in hospitals to advise during functional testing, fitting of prostheses, and prescribing of occupational therapy. The vocational department would also direct course preparation and selection of instructors, choice of occupation for the individual (in consultation with the Medical Department), and job placement of the disabled.[49]

Similarly, the surgeon general's rehabilitation plan was published as a Senate Document through a resolution introduced by the Committee on Military Affairs.[50] The report laid out the military medical plan in exact detail, down to the dimensions of workshops and kinds of apparatus to be used. The surgeon general viewed the choice of occupation for the disabled as a medical decision and stated that the individual must remain in the military for the duration of his training. He also argued that existing civilian institutions were not adequately equipped for the special needs of the disabled and that special schools in military hospitals were necessary.[51] The report stressed that training should begin in the hospital during the early stage of convalescence, as had the Federal Board when it called for the use of civilian vocational experts in hospitals. This recommendation sought to avoid fragmentation by keeping the program in the surgeon general's office "where it rightfully belongs." To placate other interests, the report suggested the establishment of an advisory board to represent all opinions.[52]

At this point, the two sides each moved to obtain legislation that would confer the authority and funds to pursue this work. The medical interests, represented by the surgeon general, staked a claim to control the total reconstruction and rehabilitation process, which would include vocational training and placement as well as "curative" work performed during recuperation. These activities had never before been claimed by any organized group of medical practitioners. On the other side, the Federal Board for Vocational Education successfully questioned the surgeon general's authority to proceed, and countered with its own plan. Implementation of this plan would have checked the expansion of the medical profession and introjected an outside authority into decisions about the physical status of patients. This intrusion was, not surprisingly, contested by medical interests.

These conflicting interests were represented at a conference called by the secretary of war in January 1918. Fifteen organizations participated, including military and federal government departments and private groups such as the American Red Cross, the American Federation of Labor, the National Manufacturers Association, and the AMA.[53] A committee was formed to reconcile varied interests, resulting in a compromise that drew a sharp distinction between medical and vocational programs by explicitly placing control over all "functional and mental restoration" in the hands of the surgeon general. Any workshops or training to accomplish this task would be considered medical and surgical work. When this phase was completed, the patient would be discharged to a proposed civilian board composed of representatives from the War Department, Navy, Department of Labor, and the Federal Board for Vocational Education. This board would control vocational rehabilitation and would advise vocational officers on the surgeon general's staff but not medical personnel. A tentative draft of a bill based on these recommendations was written and it served as the basis for a bill introduced to the Senate.[54]

This conference checked the aspirations of the Federal Board to place their vocational experts in hospitals and of the surgeon general to build hospitals to provide the full range of services under military medical control. As things stood, the surgeon general protected his own territory. He also prevented the Federal Board from gaining sole control of vocational rehabilitation by virtue of the control vested in the recommended board composed of different departments interested in this work. However, the Federal Board and its allies prevented the surgeon general's office from gaining complete control of the program and extending the boundaries of medical practice.

Before the bill was introduced in Congress, the surgeon general's plans were further set back by the White House and the Council on National Defense, which opposed the creation of a new administrative board and therefore gave control of the program to the Federal Board for Vocational Education.[55] At hearings before the Joint Committee on Education and Labor held from April 30 to May 2, 1918, the surgeon general offered support for this bill if military authority in the hospital were not threatened.[56] This signaled his failure to gain control of the program beyond the work of physical reconstruction.

The vocational rehabilitation bill was further changed in committee to limit military authority to physical restoration of the disabled. In the Senate, the debate focused on the issue of control. Two senators who were physicians led the opposition to the bill and maintained that the surgeon general had already begun a program and should be in control.[57] They were especially concerned about the possibility of interference with medical authority in the hospital.[58] Senator Smith, as sponsor of the bill, replied that there was a "certain degree of mistaken desire on the part of a surgeon to do what did not belong to his province at all and in which he has had no special experience.[59] He also noted that the surgeon general had not been granted legal authority to carry on his work in rehabilitation.[60] After a few modifications and repeated assurances that there would be no interference with military medical authority (e.g., the physician could request advice from the civilian vocational agent but did not have to do so), the opposition conceded and there was a unanimous vote in favor of the bill.[61]

The signing of the bill in July 1918 ended the surgeon general's attempt to extend the scope of medical practice to include vocational training and placement. The Medical Department, however, had been granted the exclusive right to all aspects of functional restoration and medical control over curative work brought occupational therapy into medicine's domain. The department also blocked the Federal Board for Vocational Education from gaining the legal requirement that their experts must be consulted during the hospital restoration process, although the law specified that vocational experts would be available to offer advice if requested. In fact, the department never requested such aid, and actually prohibited Federal Board representatives from entering military hospitals. Continuity of care had been espoused by all parties, but in practice the surgeon general prevented any civilian incursion on the military medical domain. The result of the standoff between the Medical Department and the Federal Board was that a sharp line had been drawn between "medical" and "vocational" rehabilitation; this was carried over to the civilian sphere with the passing of the Vocational Rehabilitation Law in 1920. Since medical services were not mentioned in this law, the two fields developed independently between the wars. Institutional means to bridge the gap between them were not provided until World War II and the 1943 Vocational Rehabilitation Law.

Resolution of external conflict with the Federal Board was accompanied by decreased conflict between medical segments. Four days after the close of the congressional hearings, the secretary of war moved to end the struggles with the Federal Board for Vocational Education and between the segments of the profession. He limited the scope of reconstruction work to physical restoration and changed the name of the division to the Division of Physical Reconstruction. Omission of the words "Special Hospitals" signified the end of plans to build reconstruction hospitals. In reference to internal conflicts, the secretary of war returned to their own services the representatives from concerned clinical specialties assigned to the division in August 1917. Furthermore, the ambiguity over who should supervise reconstruction aides ended by transferring aides in the Division of Orthopedic Surgery to the Division of Physical Reconstruction.[62]

While the secretary of war's intervention resolved much of the internal conflict over program control, the issue of which specialty would control the diagnosis and treatment of patients remained. The policy, based on the secretary of war's recommendations, was that clinical officers would diagnose and prescribe occupational and physical therapy, and educational and physiotherapeutic officers would carry out treatment.[63] Thus, for example, physiotherapy officers working under Granger in the physiotherapy section were only to follow the instructions of other physicians. The ambivalence of physiotherapists toward this situation is reflected in Granger's statement to the 1918 meeting of the American Association of Electro-Therapeutics and Radiology. In accordance with prevailing policy, he began by saying that teamwork would be the watchword and that the ward surgeon's instructions would be followed by the physiotherapist even if he disagreed with them. But Granger went on to say that the physiotherapeutic officer would call for a consultation if he felt there were contraindications to the prescribed treatment. Granger concluded his statement on a contradictory note, saying, "In most cases, however, the prescription is left to the judgment of the physiotherapeutic officer."[64]

By the end of World War I, physiotherapists achieved a formal administrative position in the Medical Department of the Army. They carved out an area where they alone would practice. However, to avoid threatening other interests in the profession, they rejected any right to make diagnoses and defined their role as supportive, in the manner of laboratory work.[65] Having received a cold reception from the surgeon general to their late entry in the competition for a share of the wartime medical market, the physiotherapists did not become actively involved in the struggles described above for control within the army; their main concern was getting the army to use their methods. Once this goal was achieved, the attention of physiotherapists turned to their position in the profession's vertical division of labor. Deprived of the right to control diagnosis and treatment, they became "technicians" for the rest of the profession.

Efforts to gain control over patient decisions resulted in a more favorable position for the physiotherapists after the war. The surgeon general granted physiotherapeutic officers the right to use their own judgment when treating patients with their methods.[66] Control over diagnosis and treatment, however, continued to be contested and renegotiated in civilian hospitals after the war and remains an unsettled issue today. One way physiotherapists could gain more control over clinical decisions was to create a corps of assistants to carry out treatment. By delegating much of their work the physiotherapists could devote more time to diagnosis, as well as to research and teaching. In this manner, they could claim special expertise based on knowledge they alone possessed, thus giving them equal standing with other specialists.

The Origins of the Allied Occupations

Physical Therapy

Prior to World War I physicians mainly relied on nurses for assistance. But some orthopedic surgeons in the Boston area used women trained in physical education, corrective exercise, and massage as assistants in their private offices.[67] Additional training given by orthopedic surgeons made it possible for these assistants to work with crippled children, especially those suffering from poliomyelitis.[68] Physiotherapists also used assistants, but because there were no effective controls these former assistants often became competitors in the fee-for-service market.[69]

Planning for war, Goldthwait, director of the orthopedic preparedness committee, called on his own assistant to organize women to do this work in the military. Other orthopedic surgeons recruited their former assistants to serve. These assistants, or women's auxiliary aides, were first placed in late 1917 in the Division of Orthopedic Surgery and specialized in application of physical agents, occupational therapy, and dietetics. Following the failure of orthopedic surgeons to control all physical reconstruction in the military, these women were renamed reconstruction physiotherapy aides and were transferred in 1918 to Granger's physiotherapy section in the newly formed Division of Physical Reconstruction.[70] This transfer firmly established a connection between the aides and physiotherapists.

Soon demand arose for these aides in army hospitals both in the United States and overseas. A special appeal was issued to colleges and physical education schools, and intensive courses, varying from six weeks to three months, were created to increase the number of civilian assistants available to the military.[71] Women accepted into these programs were usually physical education teachers with some background in anatomy. The first of these courses was organized at Walter Reed Hospital in Washington, D.C. Fourteen colleges and schools of physical education quickly established similar courses to meet requirements outlined by the surgeon general's office, the largest of which was the program at Reed College in Oregon. Further specialized training was given by Harvard University to eighty-five of the "best equipped" aides.[72]

In June 1918 the first overseas unit of reconstruction aides was ordered to France and soon these "rubbing angels," as they were known to soldiers, were scattered throughout forty-seven hospitals.[73] Although nearly 800 physiotherapy aides eventually served in the military, their specific duties remained unclear. *Carry On*, a magazine published through the Division of Physical Reconstruction, described their work as "military massage and muscle reeducation."[74] Even some commanding officers in Europe did not know what to do with these "Belgian war widows," frequently confusing them with nurses, social workers, Wacs, Waves, or "daughters of the rich."[75]

More important for the future of the occupation, the military experience created a nucleus for postwar organization by bringing together a large number of previously isolated women. Besides forming these initial communication links and social bonds, the military experience proved significant after the war.[76] Army channels were used to send over 300 letters to former reconstruction aides and orthopedic surgeons about a proposed national association.

Thus, the basis for organization among reconstruction aides was provided by war need and the Medical Department's authority to create occupational roles. These early physiotherapy aides never questioned the supervision of their work by physicians in private offices and in the Medical Department of the Army, or even later when they organized their association. Far from being the nonphysician competitors of orthopedic surgeons and physiotherapists, they were a group of assistants nurtured by physicians, who would later exchange autonomy for occupational recognition by the medical profession.

Occupational Therapy

In contrast to physical therapy, occupational therapy had a longer and more complex history as well as a more autonomous status before the war. Occupational therapists trace their roots to ancient Egypt, where a connection had been made between activity and recovery from sickness. The discipline's modern foundations are linked to the eighteenth-century European development of work therapy for mental asylum patients.[77] In the United States, such "moral treatment" or "ergotherapy" was used during the first half of the nineteenth century. After a decline following the Civil War, the field revived at the turn of the century.[78] Work was now seen as a cure for physical as well as mental infirmities rather than as a mere diversional activity.

Shortly before the United States entered World War I, several people active in this revival decided to form a professional association. In 1914, George Barton, an architect and tuberculosis patient who discovered that manual activities helped his convalescence, founded Consolation House in Clifton Springs, New York, to serve as a school, workshop, and vocational bureau for convalescing patients referred by local physicians. A year later, William Dunton, a psychiatrist interested in work as a cure for mental patients, published *Occupational Therapy, a Manual for Nurses*. After Barton read this book he approached Dunton to explore the possibility of establishing an association. Along with a nurse and a social worker interested in the recuperative effects of crafts and work, Barton and Dunton met at Consolation House in March 1917 and formed the National Society for the Promotion of Occupational Therapy.[79]

Although Barton became the society's first president, the most important influences in the profession's early years were the social worker, Eleanor Slagle, and the psychiatrist, Dunton. Dunton created a forum for communication through his editorship of the *Maryland Psychiatric Quarterly*, which all members received.[80] More important, Dunton established the tradition of occupational therapists working under physicians.[81] The adoption of a medical model was clear in Dunton's writings and in the society's constitution, which called for "the advancement of occupation as a therapeutic measure, the study of the effects of occupation upon the human being, and the dissemination of scientific knowledge of this subject."[82] Dunton quickly gained support from psychiatrists, orthopedists, neurologists, and general practitioners for the necessity of a physician's prescription and/or referral for patients receiving occupational therapy.[83] The occupational therapist would then carry out the actual therapy. In the same way physicians rely upon nurses to give medication, claimed Dunton, "so must he rely upon the therapists to administer the practical part of occupational therapy. . . . The occupational therapist, therefore, has the same relation to the physician as has the nurse, that is, she is a technical assistant."[84]

Serving as the society's second president, Dunton also

started a long-standing reliance on the medical profession for leadership. Such medical leadership was necessary, according to a statement given at the society's fiftieth anniversary, because "the infant association needed the prestige of persons closely connected with and highly esteemed by members of the medical profession in order to ensure its recognition."[85] Four of the first seven presidents of the national association were physicians, and the eighth, though not a physician, was managing director of the National Board of Medical Examiners. Thus, "for the first thirty years of its existence the Association was led by men, except for Mrs. Slagle, who were persons of such recognized qualifications and reputation."[86]

Members of the society formed a preparedness committee in 1917 to press for the inclusion of occupational therapy in the surgeon general's war programs and to convince the medical profession that their methods were useful. At first, this effort was met by "a wall of reactionary medical and military opposition."[87] Even a base officer's request for occupational therapists to serve in Europe was rejected because the military could not understand that he wanted a program of vocational training rather than basket weaving.[88] Persistence led, in 1918, to the appointment of occupational therapists to the corps of reconstruction aides and a request by the surgeon general for a thousand of these women.[89] Short training courses, emphasizing crafts for recreation and rehabilitation, were created to meet the new demand for therapists.[90] By the war's end there were only 116 "ill-trained, enthusiastic ladies" to develop a crafts program to rehabilitate the wounded.[91]

Caught up in the wartime struggle over vocational rehabilitation, occupational therapists attempted to extend the boundaries of their field to include not only the early diversional and more recent curative uses of work activity but also vocational education. They argued that "vocational training or education per se is not a form of occupational therapy, but when given to reestablish function, to give more normal view of life, it may well be classed as a form of occupational therapy."[92]

The future position of occupational therapy in the rehabilitation division of labor depended on the struggle between medicine and vocational education for program control. The willingness of the surgeon general to accept occupational therapy reflected its potential to bridge the medical and vocational aspects of rehabilitation. The basis of occupational therapy, convalescent curative work, fell between the acute care stage, in which diversional activities were used, and the vocational reeducation phase, which was contested.

The result of the military medical interests' failure to control the vocational aspect of rehabilitation was that occupational therapy was also checked in its attempt to include vocational education within its boundaries. The question of where therapeutic use of work ended and practical teaching of work-related skills began would not emerge again until World War II, when renewed medical involvement in rehabilitation brought occupational therapy and its relationship to vocational rehabilitation to the fore.

However, in the debate over the boundaries of medical and vocational aspects of rehabilitation during World War I, medicine's claim that work should be prescribed only by a physician was not questioned by the Federal Board for Vocational Education or by the fledgling occupational therapy association.[93] Occupational therapy, which defined itself as the "science of healing by occupation," had been placed squarely in the medical camp. Lack of medical involvement in postwar vocational rehabilitation led to a decline of interest in occupational therapy until World War II.

The Impact of War

The war aroused patriotic sentiments expressed in the image of a wounded and permanently disabled soldier. To see wounded soldiers safely crossing a street is "a wonderful sight," said an article in *Carry On*, "indeed the people in the taxis and limousines seemed proud that . . . they could show these men how glad they were to wait for them as they slowly hobbled over the pavement. A limp arm in khaki—ah! how noble it looks!"[94] Government and private organizations, like the U.S. Public Health Service and the American

Red Cross, moved rapidly to support new programs to rehabilitate soldiers as part of our "national debt" and speed their reentrance into civilian life.[95] These organizations sensed an opportunity to extend disability programs after the war to industrial accident victims and to chronically ill patients. The war also changed the division of labor in medicine and the future of occupations within it. Rapid increase in the demand for medical services and the involvement of individuals from emerging specialties in the Medical Department of the Army encouraged such innovation. Attempts by these individuals to control some portion of the military medical program resulted in competition among segments and the creation of new occupational roles.

The most important consequence of the war for physiotherapists was their institutionalization in the Medical Department of the Army and the legitimacy this gave them. Despite difficulties in controlling their work, this legitimacy bolstered the status of what, prior to the war, had been a segment whose position was becoming increasingly uncertain. The war also marked the first time physical modes of treatment were focused specifically on injuries and chronic disabilities. And, finally, the physiotherapists and other segments lost control over rehabilitation to the Federal Board for Vocational Education, which became responsible for civilian rehabilitation in 1920.

Without public support for medical services in rehabilitation, organized physiotherapists returned to seeking acceptance of their methods for the treatment of a wide variety of acute and chronic problems. Owing to the war experience, the medical profession's skepticism toward the simpler physical therapies declined.[96] The successful use of hydrotherapy, massage, and exercise with wounded soldiers led some medical authorities to conclude that "physical therapy is of great value," and "its scope is wide."[97] Electrotherapy, however, remained a marginal practice in the eyes of medicine.[98] The eventual demise in the 1930s of the American Association of Electro-Therapeutics and Radiology resulted from its persistent emphasis on medical electricity.

The war also led to the creation of a new occupation and the extension of an existing one. Control over wartime organizational mechanisms allowed a small group of physicians to rapidly enact on a large scale what they had done for years in private practice. The role of physiotherapy aide was created, even though nurses already provided the major source of assistance to physicians. Nurses found it difficult to meet the increasing demand for acute care, which they defined as their work, but they were also unwilling to reduce their "cherished standards" so that the supply of practitioners could be increased. Finally forced to do this, they bemoaned the destruction of the line between "nurse" and "untrained" worker. As nurses saw it, the dilemma was to meet the demand or face the introduction of short courses that would undermine standards.[99]

Because nurses continued to define their work as acute care and to resist the lowering of standards, physicians in the surgeon general's office never seriously considered using nurses to assist in the application of physical agents. Also, assistants used by Boston physicians before the war usually had a physical education background; planning for new reconstruction aides reflected this precedent. This was so even though, until World War II, many physical therapists were first trained as nurses, and struggles for control over physiotherapy departments developed between nurses and physical therapists. While nurses were at first uninterested in physical therapeutics and rehabilitation work with wounded soldiers, as indicated by the absence of such issues in the *American Journal of Nursing,* they later desired control of these new hospital workers. The creation of rehabilitation nursing after World War II reflected the changing view of nurses toward this work.

Thus, rapid escalation of demand, occupational rigidity and lack of interest, and control over an administrative apparatus led to the establishment of what later became physical therapy. The war also proved significant for other occupations that would eventually enter the rehabilitation field. We saw how occupational therapy organized on the basis of a claim about the therapeutic effects of work, and how its relationship to rehabilitation led to incorporation by the Medical Department of the Army. This involvement in the military linked the future of occupational therapy with the medical profession. Two other groups would become part of the division of labor in medical rehabilitation. At the request of the Council on National Defense, the makers of artificial limbs met in Washington in 1917 and organized the Association of Artificial Limb Manufacturers of the United States.[100] In a blend of the "commercial" and the "professional," this association specified standards, training, and certification for workers in the field of orthotics and prosthetics. Also, a section for the treatment of speech and hearing defects was established in the Medical Department, where training was given to teachers and corrective speech workers.[101] Originally created as a specialty for speech teachers, speech therapy spun off as a separate occupation in the 1920s and became an integral part of medical rehabilitation after World War II. However, the medical profession and the specialty of rehabilitation medicine have failed in their attempts to control speech therapy.

In short, World War I greatly influenced the setting of occupational boundaries and the organization of medical services. These changes in the structure of work were to have long-range implications for the future division of labor in the field of medical rehabilitation.

4

Foundations for a Division of Labor, 1920–1941

The nineteenth-century medical market had been competitive and sectarian. In the twentieth century, the regular medical profession's gain of exclusive rights to certain tasks eliminated many medical sects and healers. Those nonphysician practitioners who remained had their services legally delimited, although osteopaths and chiropractors were still competitors. While the number of different groups providing medical care was declining, the internal complexity of the medical profession was increasing. By the early 1920s more than twenty segments existed in the profession. Interested groups contested control of these segments and how they should be differentiated. Licensing, training, and professional certification were all considered. The outcome of this contest resulted in the demarcation of specialty boundaries.[1]

In this struggle, the AMA favored university-based specialty education, thereby undercutting the influence of specialty organizations. The AMA appointed fifteen committees representing various specialties to investigate education in each area. These committees became the locus for specialty conflict and were the forerunners of the specialty boards established in the 1930s. Two AMA councils also created a precedent for intervention in specialty affairs during the 1920s.

The Council on Medical Education and Hospitals became the accrediting body for laboratories and radiology departments, and the Council on Physical Therapy was to control the manufacture of physical therapy equipment. Yet in this decade the segments remained autonomous, thwarting the AMA.

This autonomy ended in the early 1930s when a coalition of groups formed the Advisory Board for Medical Specialties to recognize certain segments as specialties and to determine entry standards. Although the AMA withdrew from this board, its Council on Medical Education and Hospitals worked behind the scenes to develop the "Essentials for an Approved Special Examining Board." The AMA and the advisory board thus achieved some control over the granting of specialty status to segments. By the late 1930s almost all segments desired such status.

Physical Therapy Physicians Between the Wars

Professional Developments

After the war, physicians specializing in physical modes of treatment changed their name from physiotherapists to "physical therapy physicians." Despite wartime interest in rehabilitation, they soon returned to acute care medicine, which they had largely practiced before the war. The omission of medical services in the 1920 civilian Vocational Rehabilitation Law meant that physical therapy physicians would not be reimbursed for rehabilitating disabled and chronically ill patients. Therefore they continued to advocate their prewar position; their skills were for the diagnosis and cure of a wide variety of medical problems.

Physical therapy physicians' curative perspective toward acute diseases was most apparent in the key physical therapy journal, *Archives of Physical Therapy*. From 1920 to 1940 only two articles in the *Archives* referred to rehabilitation, and neither was written by a physical therapy physician. In fact, the authors were from the potentially competitive specialties of industrial medicine and orthopedic surgery.[2] There were also very few publications in the *Archives* on disabling and chronic conditions. Many problems currently treated by the field, including back pain, spastic disease, stroke, spinal cord injury, and amputation, were completely ignored by the journal. When problems such as arthritis received attention, the article's focus was almost always curative rather than rehabilitative. Clearly, then, publications in the *Archives* reveal no major shift from curing acute diseases to rehabilitating chronic conditions. Reformulation of the ideology underlying physical therapy medicine did not begin until World War II, at which time the rehabilitation of chronic and disabling conditions was made the basis of the field.

Important organizational developments, however, did occur in the 1920s and 1930s. The recently formed Radiological Society of North America began publication of the *Journal of Radiology* in 1920. Infighting and policy disputes between Dr. Albert Tyler, the editor and owner of the journal, and other Radiological Society members led the society in 1923 to publish *Radiology* as its official publication. Tyler continued publishing the *Journal of Radiology* and claimed it was the Radiological Society's official organ. In the same year Tyler and several other radiologists formed the American College of Radiology and Physiotherapy to act as a "clearing house" for smaller physiotherapy and radiology organizations. Tyler soon severed ties with the Radiological Society and moved to align the *Journal of Radiology* with the college. After losing a court case to block further publication of *Radiology*, he formalized ties to the college and changed the journal's name in 1925 to the *Archives of Physical Therapy, X-Ray, Radium*.

The eventual loss of the x-ray to radiologists was symbolized in 1925 by the association's change of name to the American College of Physical Therapy, and in 1929 to the American Congress of Physical Therapy. This new, midwestern-based organization and the older American Association of Electro-Therapeutics and Radiology, renamed the American Physical Therapy Association in 1929, both represented the interests of physiotherapy during the rest of the 1920s. Increasing financial difficulties during the Depression led the American

Physical Therapy Association to merge with the American Congress of Physical Therapy in 1932, although the latter maintained its identity and control. The names of the journals published by each of the organizations were also combined to form the *Archives of Physical Therapy, X-Ray, Radium: A Journal of Physical Therapeutics*. The *Archives*, however, continued to publish articles on the use of x-rays and radium, and did not omit these technologies from its title until 1938.[3]

The Battle Against Competitors

Physical therapy physicians faced competition in the fee-for-service market and in the hospital. The most useful strategy with internal competitors in the open market was to convince the profession and individual practitioners that physical therapy was useful and to attack heroic medicine. They enlisted AMA support to eliminate external competitors by closing their schools and passing laws to restrict their practices. For the most part, though, physical therapy physicians avoided struggles with competitors in specific institutional spheres.

Physical therapy physicians were more successful at limiting competition in the open market than in hospitals because their standing had improved in the profession. In 1923 the AMA passed a resolution calling for recognition of special medical activities such as physical and occupational therapy and the "science of radiology" as integral parts of medicine and surgery.[4] More important, in 1925 the AMA formed the Council on Physical Therapy to curb claims made by manufacturers of physical therapy devices and to promote the proper use of physical therapy methods. Indeed, the editor of *JAMA* estimated that at least one hundred different companies made electrotherapeutic apparatus alone, and that countless other firms sold physical therapy equipment.[5] These "things were being advertised with unjust claims," and "exaggerations were the basis of most physical therapeutic literature."[6] The council later became the primary exponent of physical therapy methods in the AMA.

The council's first report, in 1926, noted the gradual acceptance of physical therapy but warned against "bad habits" leading to quackery and commercial abuses. The report maintained that physical therapy should be used with drugs and surgery but never as the sole treatment. As an adjunct to other forms of treatment, the report noted, physical therapy should only be prescribed by a physician trained in this area. The greatest concern of the report was with nonmedical practitioners of physical therapy. It strongly recommended that physicians not refer patients to these improperly trained "charlatans" and, further, that physicians discourage them from establishing private practices.[7]

The report expressed concern over the "unscrupulous so-called 'physio-therapist'"[8] for several reasons. These practitioners were seen as deceiving patients because they treated "imaginary ailments" with useless machines. When physiotherapy was practiced this way, especially in places such as barbershops or athletic clubs, the field received "an undeserved black eye among many medical men who are thoroughly disgusted with so much commercialism."[9] Irregular practitioners of physiotherapy were also seen as "serious" competitors for patients. According to one of the presidents of the American Congress of Physical Therapy, all "quacks" practicing physiotherapy in California earned a total of over one hundred million dollars a year while regular physicians earned far less.[10]

The council's first few years were devoted to setting standards for infrared and ultraviolet generators, sunlamps, diathermy apparatus, shoes, surgical belts, hearing aids, exercising machines, electric blankets, anesthesia equipment, and ophthalmological devices. Manufacturers were asked to send their new equipment to the council for inspection. Cooperating with physicists, engineers, and physicians, the council examined 356 pieces of apparatus by the mid-1930s and rejected almost half of these "since they obviously revealed no therapeutic efficacy."[11]

The creation of physical therapy departments in hospitals gave the field increased legitimacy by the 1930s. This led to a second report by the council in 1936. By this time the AMA had shifted its policy to one endorsing specialty formation. Reflecting this change, the report observed that physical therapy was no longer relegated to an adjunct role in treatment. Although "physical therapy is a smaller and less developed field than either medicine or surgery . . . it is possible to conceive of instances in which the use of some physical measure will be the primary method of treatment and medical agents or surgical procedures may be the adjunct."[12] However, physical therapy physicians were warned not to usurp the diagnostic prerogative of primary physicians.

The report voiced fewer fears about technicians and other nonmedical practitioners because physicians were establishing greater control over them. "Educational" efforts by the American Congress of Physical Therapy and the Council on Physical Therapy of the AMA increased the reluctance of physicians to refer to these practitioners. In addition, a number of court cases blocked efforts by "quacks" or "cultists" to gain protective licensing legislation. For example, the *Archives of Physical Therapy* called attention to a bill sponsored by the Massage Operators Guild in California which would "legalize a body of rubbers" and give them the right to control hydrotherapy. The bill was characterized as a dangerous precedent to the health of the citizenry and it was eventually defeated.[13] In another case hailed as an important ruling, the Arizona Supreme Court upheld the conviction of a naturopath who used a diathermy apparatus to burn a growth he diagnosed as cancer. The court ruled that this constituted illegal practice of surgery. The editor of the *Archives* pointed to the necessity for such legal protection for all physical therapy measures, and for the support of all those "interested in the scientific advancement of physical therapy . . . to overcome ignorance and avarice for the protection of the patient and our profession."[14] The outcome of cases such as these gave physical therapy physicians the protective umbrella sought for years against competition from nonmedical practitioners.

Competition from technicians was a more complex problem. Specialists like pathologists, radiologists, anesthesiologists, and physical therapy physicians provided technical and supportive services, which meant that some physicians viewed them as mere "technicians" and elected to use their nonphysician competitors. To reduce this competition, they tried to convince the AMA that referrals to technicians should be stopped. Physical therapy physicians claimed that technicians had "limited qualifications" and were "in direct competition with the orthodox practice of medicine. Unfortunately such a competition . . . is actually depriving legitimate physicians of a clientele which by every moral and human law should be theirs."[15] The AMA, however, was reluctant to proscribe referrals to external practitioners because other physicians wanted to retain such referral rights. The result was that competition in the open market was reinforced for physical therapy physicians and their role in hospitals was threatened.

The council's 1926 report did not distinguish between cultists and technicians in condemning the practice of "many physicians [who] may refer patients to technicians—masseurs, gymnasts, or nurses who have received training in physical therapy, or even to members of various cults for physical therapeutic treatment."[16] Yet physical therapy physicians were quick to point out that "ethical technicians" should not be confused with the "second group of poorly trained technicians with no ideals except to make money—many of these are running individual offices where they treat patients even though not referred by physicians."[17] The 1936 report sought to "elaborate on this . . . by commenting that there are ethical technicians in the field who work in various hospitals and institutional departments under the direction of physicians and occasionally as technical assistants specializing in the field."[18]

Physical therapy physicians did not want to eliminate trained technicians, as the first report implied. They only wanted to keep technicians out of fee-for-service, private practice and under the supervision of physicians so they would not be competitors in the open market. To do this, physical therapy physicians did not try to limit technician competition through the legal process, as was done with cultists. They instead sought to control technicians and to develop a structured hospital relationship with them which would preserve a role for the physical therapy physician.

The American Congress of Physical Therapy and the AMA Council on Medical Education and Hospitals established for-

mal relations in 1934 with the American Physiotherapy Association, which represented technicians. The congress was
empowered to create and maintain a registry of technicians
who met designated standards, while the council was to accredit technician schools. Physical therapy technicians in return agreed that their work should be supervised and
prescribed by physicians. Acceptance of the title "technician"
symbolized this subordination: technicians previously called
themselves physical therapists or physiotherapists.[19]

In the late 1930s physical therapy physicians became increasingly concerned with their place in the hospital. Although they were involved in the struggles over military
medical programs and patient care during the war, physical
therapy physicians paid little attention to issues of organizational power and control in the years following. There were,
of course, some exceptions. For example, one prominent person in the field wrote in 1922 that physical therapy physicians
should direct physical therapy departments in hospitals and
control the prescribing of treatment. In this view, the primary
care physician would merely request physical therapy services
and a desired outcome, rather than suggest a specific treatment.[20] In general, however, physical therapy physicians
seemed unconcerned about this issue after the war. Instead
they again tried to improve their status in the fee-for-service
market by gaining general acceptance for physical therapy
methods. Efforts to change their position in hospitals would
contradict this goal by implying an interest in the specialty
status they eschewed. As a result, most hospitals established
physical therapy departments with orthopedic surgeons or
technicians in charge.[21]

As physical therapy physicians pushed for specialty status
in the late 1930s, this situation became more important to
them. Concern over their hospital role relative to that of technicians was exemplified by an editorial in the *Archives*. The
editor attacked a recent article by a physician who suggested
that anyone could give physical therapy treatment and that
it was thus not necessary for a physician trained in these
techniques to be involved in hospital physical therapy departments. The editor responded by stressing the need for a
physician specializing in physical therapy to supervise this

work. Drawing on the analogy that drugs were not entrusted to a pharmaceutical apprentice, the editor maintained that improper use of physical therapy measures could be just as dangerous. Also, the editor held that the role of the technician should correspond to that of the nurse, and that if the technician did not follow the orders of physicians trained in physical therapy "medical anarchy" would result. Emphasizing the difficulty of this work, the editor stated that heat did not involve just the use of a hot water bottle, but the application of a complicated apparatus which required more than simply "turning a switch." Similarly, massage was described as a "highly developed art," and "the art and science of exercise [as being] more complicated and difficult to learn and apply than pharmaco-therapy."[22]

The maintenance of a role in hospitals required physical therapy physicians to change their earlier strategy. Rather than persuading others to use their methods, they now claimed that only they were competent to perform certain tasks. Although physicians could perform basic physical therapy techniques, more difficult procedures required specialists. This position was elaborated in Krusen's 1938 presidential address to the American Congress of Physical Therapy. "The attitude of those who insist that physical therapy is not a specialty is fallacious," argued Krusen. "While it is true that there are many forms of physical therapy which are elaborate and which require highly trained individuals for their administration, there are also many simple physical measures which should be used by all physicians."[23] He placed physical therapy in a situation analogous to that of pathology where simple tests like blood counts were done by general practitioners, while the laboratory was used for more complex tests.

Krusen and others in the field created a second professional association in 1938 specifically to pursue this new strategy. The Society of Physical Therapy Physicians met the guidelines established by the Advisory Board for Medical Specialties. Membership was restricted to physicians in academic or equivalent positions with five years experience in physical therapy.[24] Thus, physical therapy physicians maintained two separate professional organizations to conduct different strategies. The ideology of simple techniques performed by all and difficult ones performed only by specialists in the field linked these two goals. Although the ideology and purposes of the organizations have changed somewhat, this dual organizational structure still exists today.

Before World War II physical therapy physicians were more preoccupied with competition from technicians than from other specialists occupying important positions in physical therapy departments. This preoccupation reflected their immediate concern that physicians rather than technicians head such departments. Without this precedent there would be no role for physical therapy physicians in the hospital. Although some departments were headed by other specialists, overt conflict with physical therapy physicians was rare.

There was also little conflict with orthopedic surgeons, despite their relationship to physical therapy technicians. In addition to heading physical therapy departments and using physical therapy technicians in their own practices, orthopedic surgeons developed advisory relationships with the associations representing physical therapy technicians and occupational therapists.[25] Generally, orthopedists conceived of physical therapy as the "handmaiden of every branch of medicine" and, more specificially, as an adjunct to orthopedic surgery.[26] Only after physical therapy physicians established that it was necessary for a physician to direct physical therapy departments did they turn their attention to competition from other specialties and to the control of these departments. Once again, these conflicts occurred in the context of wartime opportunity.

The Allied Occupations: Institutionalization and Subordination

Physical Therapy

Harold Corbusier, a physical therapy physician, first proposed a national organization for World War I physiotherapy aides. During the war Corbusier helped organize the orthopedic surgery section in the surgeon general's office and observed the successful use of reconstruction aides in the military.[27] Shortly after the war ended Corbusier wrote to Mary McMillan, a leading aide, that an organization of aides could "advertise to the physicians and surgeons of the country the importance of the various methods of treatment of physical means." He also hoped the association would "elevate and standardize the work and place it on a more substantial basis [and] . . . urge upon the various hospitals the importance of establishing departments of physiotherapy."[28] Corbusier's letter suggests that physical therapy physicians thought such an organization would aid their campaign to gain the medical profession's acceptance of physical therapy.

In 1921 thirty former military aides and six physicians met in New York City and organized the American Women's Physical Therapeutic Association. Among the physicians was Granger, former chief of the surgeon general's physical therapy section and past president of the American Association of Electro-Therapeutics and Radiology. The name of the new organization was soon changed to the American Physiotherapy Association (APA) and membership was opened to all. Admission to the association required candidates to be "graduates of schools of physiotherapy or physical education, who have had training and experience in massage and therapeutic exercise, with some knowledge of either electrotherapy or hydrotherapy." The omission of nurses was quickly challenged and the constitution was changed to allow those with nursing backgrounds to become members. The new association, however, opposed any attempt to place physical therapy technicians under the supervision of nurses. In one case, for example, aides in an army hospital protested a plan to put nurses in charge of the physical therapy department and the association successfully pressured the surgeon general to rescind the plan.

In its early years, the APA published a journal, held annual conferences, and attempted to raise standards. By the late 1920s the association moved to set standards and accredit schools in response to the threat posed by the growing number of untrained technicians used in physicians' offices and hospitals. It was "deplorable," claimed an editorial in the *Physiotherapy Review*, that so many offices and hospitals "refer to the commercial house that supplied their apparatus to supply a technician, whose only knowledge of the treatment of disease is a short course in electrotherapy."[29] Another editorial in the same journal expressed such outrage at the hiring of "inefficiently trained assistants" by physicians that it singled out one such correspondence school for attack. A particular cause for the outrage was the school's advertising "physiotherapy as the easier way to greater income, a simple way to solve the problem of more money. No advance education is necessary: ability to read and write and to understand simple instruction is all that is required."[30] The association, however, did not have any legal means to enforce standards or accredit schools. Inability to regulate its own affairs eventually led to formalization of the association's subordinate status to the legally powerful medical profession.

The first constitution of the association briefly mentioned its relationship to medicine. While one of the association's goals was to "make available efficiently trained women to the medical profession," nothing was said about only working under the direction of physicians. This qualification was later added to the third constitution, which stated, "we must . . . stick to our own field, which is the carrying out of prescriptions given by doctors and not diagnosing, prescribing, or in any way experimenting in the treatment of disease."[31]

This proclamation of fidelity by members of the association was not enough for physical therapy physicians. In 1924 they pressured the newly organized aides to use the title "physiotherapy technician" instead of physiotherapist. APA members rejected this request, and the controversy continued for several years. Many members, particularly some of the "mature, cultured, and highly trained women" who started the association were unwilling to be labeled technicians.[32] If they could not use the title physiotherapist, argued one member, then they should at least pick a name that clearly expressed their "professional attitude" rather than one that suggested they were "mere technicians"[33] only capable of "holding a water hose or turning on an electric switch."[34]

During this period the APA unsuccessfully sought affiliation with the AMA to distinguish itself from the cults and "drugless healers" who also claimed to practice physiotherapy. Some early members hoped to make this distinction through licensure laws. The association's legislative committee, "impressed in its travels through the East with the numerous self-named 'physiotherapists,' illiterate and untrained, working in small cities," called for each association chapter to "bend its energies toward the enactment of proper legislation for the protection of physiotherapy."[35] The association's lack of political power made this impossible and forced them to try to merely block attempts by competitors to obtain legislation. Even in this limited area, success often depended on the support of local medical societies. The association created a standing committee in 1928 to pursue this defensive role. In California, for example, the association gained the support of the state medical association and the state board of medical license to throw a bill out of committee which would have prohibited anyone from being a masseur unless trained in a school of massage.[36] The association also pressured hospitals and the medical profession not to use technicians trained in commercially based short courses. In all these activities the association sought support from organized medicine, and worked on an informal basis with the Council on Physical Therapy and the AMA Council on Medical Education and Hospitals.[37]

As it became increasingly apparent that the APA could not achieve its goals, opposition to the "technician" label declined. A 1930 editorial observed: "We shall greet this year as previously with that ever-present question, 'What's in a name?' We have grown old in debate but have never yet worn out the subject. . . . We can be 'physiotherapists' or 'physiotherapy technicians' or what have you as long as we are there."[38] This was followed by official acceptance of the "technician" title by the association, although many members continued to resent the term.[39]

Adoption of this title signaled the end of organized resistance to medical domination. The APA's efforts were now focused on increasing the demand for its members' services and formalizing its relationship with the AMA. To increase demand by physicians, the association clarified and publicized the nature of physiotherapy to the medical profession and distinguished their expertise from that of other practitioners. So confused was medicine and the laity, one association member was prompted to ask rhetorically: "What is a physiotherapist? Is it dead or alive? Is it animal, vegetable, or mineral?" Most people simply did not know the answer to this question, claimed this technician, while others had a "hazy" idea that a physiotherapist was the same as a chiropractor or masseuse.[40] Other association members thought the confusion lay in distinguishing physiotherapy from physical education.[41] The way to end this confusion, according to technicians, was to become "very conscious of the importance and need of 'selling' the American Physiotherapy Association" and "to preach and act to extend the gospel for which we stand."[42]

In 1933 a resolution submitted to the AMA House of Delegates asked the medical profession to accredit physiotherapy schools. The resolution passed, and the task of accrediting schools for physical therapy technicians was assumed by the Council on Medical Education and Hospitals with the advice and assistance of the Council on Physical Therapy. By 1936 the Council on Medical Education and Hospitals published the "Essentials of an Acceptable School for Physical Therapy Technicians" and began to inspect these schools according to the "Essentials."[43] Only thirteen of the thirty-five schools received the council's approval that year.[44]

The APA also established a formal relationship with the American Congress of Physical Therapy in 1936 to further control entry into the occupation. This control took the form of a registry of qualified individuals to be compiled by the congress. As was the case with AMA accreditation arrangements, physical therapy technicians pursued organized medicine's assistance in establishing some kind of registration system. In 1926 a representative of the association asked physicians to develop a system of state registration for physical therapy technicians,[45] but nothing was done until the American Congress of Physical Therapy created a committee to study this issue in 1933. A year later this committee published its plan in the *Archives*.

Although technicians were pleased that physicians finally responded to their requests, some expressed misgivings about having connections with only one specialty. They argued that a board responsible for setting standards should represent all specialties involved in this work. Technicians may also have been reticent to establish ties with what was still a marginal segment in the medical profession, and one that might never achieve specialty status. In the mid-1930s, when other segments were being granted such status, this may have been of major importance to technicians. In addition, technicians were suspicious of physical therapy physicians' material interests in controlling their work. Some felt that "the medical body organized to assume control over the physical therapy technicians" because of "a desire to increase its revenues."[46] The association therefore recommended that it contact the American Orthopedic Society as well as other groups.[47]

The congress acted on its committee's recommendations in 1934 and formed the American Registry of Physical Therapy Technicians. Seven congress members who exclusively practiced physical therapy were appointed to the board of the registry.[48] Since physical therapy technicians were unable to get representatives of other specialties on the board, they entered into an agreement with the supposedly autonomous American Registry of Physical Therapy Technicians. This relationship was never harmonious. Registry control was in the hands of physicians who represented the American Congress of Physical Therapy, and the participation of technicians was limited to an advisory board. Initially, the advisory board had no control over policy, so the American Physiotherapy Association pressured for a veto power requiring board approval of any proposed rules.

In addition, the registry attempted to restrict the practice of technicians by not allowing them to set up "private offices," which the American Physiotherapy Association defined as "without physician supervision." Although technicians practicing in the fee-for-service market readily accepted physician supervision, they represented competition to physical therapy physicians.[49] General practitioners and other specialists often referred their private patients to these technicians for treatment, and the AMA refused to take a strong stand against technician referrals. The *Archives* openly acknowledged this competition from physical therapy technicians in independent practice and announced that "effective measures" would be taken "to stem a movement which was sure to grow into what is perhaps best described as another pseudomedical profession."[50] Physical therapy physicians now could reduce open market competition by refusing to register individuals if they practiced in "private offices."

Open market competition from physical therapy technicians declined during the late 1930s. As noted above, the 1936 report of the AMA's Council on Physical Therapy showed less concern about technician competition than the 1926 report. The ability of the registry to control the practice of technicians had much to do with this change in attitude. Technicians' fears of becoming dependent on and subordinate to physical therapy physicians were confirmed; the connection with the American Congress of Physical Therapy was increasingly perceived as oppressive.[51]

However, physical therapy technicians did benefit from their connections to the AMA and the American Congress of Physical Therapy. First, they survived as an occupation by establishing a distinct boundary between their "legitimate" medical work and the allegedly low quality, and often dangerous, practice of cultists. Second, they acquired mechanisms to standardize the education of future members and to control entry into the occupation. In essence, they traded their ability to work in the fee-for-service market for help in structuring their position in other markets as employees of hospitals or physicians.

When an occupational group has been closed out of the fee-for-service market, adoption of the medical profession's strategy of creating an inelastic demand situation by eliminating competition and then restricting practitioner supply is no longer feasible. Rather than pursuing the legal capacity to eliminate market competitors, allied occupations seek labor market controls that permit them to articulate supply and demand factors. The key is to turn a potentially elastic demand situation into a more inelastic one by guaranteeing demand for the particular service that only their occupation can provide, and then to recruit and train enough qualified individuals to meet this demand. Demand is guaranteed by requiring institutions to employ only those persons meeting specific requirements. The result is a higher wage than would have been paid if the institution had been free to organize jobs and to hire anyone it wished to fill them.[52]

Although physical therapy technicians obtained controls over members' skills and entry into the occupation by the 1930s, these controls were not sufficient to improve their competitive economic position. Employers had to be required to hire physical therapy technicians. To do this, the technicians tried to influence organizations competing to control standardization and accreditation of hospitals. These organizations included the AMA's Council on Medical Education and Hospitals, the American Hospital Association, and the American College of Surgeons. One of the organizations, the American College of Surgeons, submitted to this pressure and required hospitals seeking a "Grade A" classification to employ only physical therapy technicians meeting the American Physiotherapy Association's standards.[53] To the extent that such accreditation requirements became important for hospitals to receive government funds and other benefits, competitors of the physical therapy technicians would be restricted from working in a portion of the market.

However, the AMA's Council on Medical Education and Hospitals rebuffed American Physiotherapy Association efforts to influence accreditation requirments. The association requested that hospitals deny employment to workers who were not members of the association or did not meet its standards.[54] In a forthright rejection of this request, one physician asserted that the council would not "meddle in the internal affairs of hospitals" and could not support the economic interests of any group.[55]

Physical therapy technicians also resisted attempts by some physicians to create a junior classification for technicians falling short of the minimum standards.[56] If these attempts had succeeded, physicians would have had a cheaper labor pool available. Physical therapy technicians were trying to raise minimum standards and successfully blocked such moves by physicians for many years. Only recently has the association, of its own volition, instituted subclassifications by level of training.

Occupational Therapy

In the early 1920s, the young but greatly expanded National Society for the Promotion of Occupational Therapy had almost five hundred members.[57] The society held annual meetings and published its own journal, the *Archives of Occupational Therapy*. In 1923 the name of the society was changed to the American Occupational Therapy Association (AOTA). Two years later the journal was renamed *Occupational Therapy and Rehabilitation*, symbolizing what was to become a predominant focus of occupational therapy.

With the return to peace, occupational therapists again complained about lack of acceptance by medicine.[58] AOTA requested its "young women" to "enlist the sympathy and the backing of the medical men . . . who either will not or cannot write the occupational therapy prescriptions."[59] Yet the association warned: "Perhaps it is too much to expect the conservative and slowly moving trend of opinion in medicine to have reached a point where occupational therapy can take its place as a definite hospital function."[60]

Despite such complaints, occupational therapists slowly extended their practice beyond mental institutions. They were readily accepted in tuberculosis sanatoriums,[61] and gained a foothold in treating industrial accident cases when the Federal Industrial Rehabilitation Act included occupational therapy as a required service.[62] They encountered greater resistance in orthopedic hospitals,[63] and especially in treating acutely ill patients in general hospitals.[64] Such resistance prompted AOTA president T. B. Kidner to express his "disappointment" that the "'carry over' to civilian orthopedic hospitals from the fine work of the army hospitals . . . seems to have been remarkably small," and that general hospitals remained "untouched" by occupational therapy.[65]

Occupational therapy's involvement with rehabilitation can be traced to Kidner, AOTA's president between 1923 and 1928. Kidner's background as an architect and an authority on the construction of institutions for the physically handicapped made him particularly well suited to plan rehabilitation services during World War I.[66] After the war, he began to connect occupational therapy's future expansion with the rehabilitation movement.[67] Patients with handicaps and orthopedic problems as well as those with general medical, surgical, and mental conditions all represented "scarcely scratched" fields "capable of very large development," claimed Kidner.[68] In a 1927 letter to William Dunton, the psychiatrist who had helped found the association, he noted the broadening scope of occupational therapy. "There is a great zone at present," wrote Kidner, "between pure occupational therapy and vocational rehabilitation which in my judgment can best be occupied and covered by occupational therapists who have the vision."[69]

Occupational therapists, like physical therapy technicians, sought to control the entry of workers, at specified levels of skill, through accreditation and certification. AOTA members were warned that they should make "certain that the back door is very carefully fastened against pretenders, that others do not crawl in under the fence, and that those who are permitted to enter the front door have the proper credentials of admission."[70] In 1935 they used the same strategy as physical therapy technicians, developing formal ties with the AMA's Council on Medical Education and Hospitals to establish a mechanism for accrediting occupational therapy schools. This alliance was heralded by occupational therapists as a sign of medical interest, and helped to raise their status and stabilize their position.[71] At the same time, they officially acknowledged their subordinate position vis-à-vis the medical profession and surrendered some autonomy.

In their other relationships, both inside and outside the medical profession, occupational therapists differed from physical therapy technicians. Their efforts to control entry culminated in an autonomous, self-regulated mechanism rather than a registry run by physicians. Minimum standards for training occupational therapists were adopted in 1923 and by 1926 the AOTA officially called for the establishment of its own national list of certified therapists.[72] Occupational therapists became increasingly committed to this self-certification mechanism as a symbol of their professionalism. "Practically everyone has had opportunity of realizing how one black sheep has affected the prestige of the white rams and ewes," stated an editorial in the association's journal. "Let us then start our registered 'flock' with *no* black sheep. At this stage again recall the occupational therapist (?) who could *only* make silk flowers."[73] It was particularly important that they did not enter into subordinating agreements with medical specialties as had physical therapy technicians with physical therapy physicians. While occupational therapists lacked specialty support, their destiny would not be determined by the needs and aspirations of a medical specialty.

Occupational therapists, unlike physical therapy technicians, did not find it necessary to surrender autonomy in return for alliance with a specialty. From medicine's viewpoint, there was little reason to establish control over occupational therapists; they were not a competitive threat, since almost all their market consisted of salaried positions in organizations. From the perspective of occupational therapy, an alliance with a specialty promised few benefits because the competition they faced was in hospitals rather than in the fee-for-service market.

Occupational therapists instead allied with the American Hospital Association (AHA), an organization that could influence hospital policies and structure. Affiliation with the AHA "makes for better feeling and understanding and the wheels of hospital administration so far as occupational therapy is concerned are apt to move less creakily."[74] This affiliation was considered so important that some members even threatened to withdraw from the association if affiliation with the AHA was discontinued.[75] The AOTA held its annual conference in conjunction with the AHA from 1923 to 1937, at AHA invitation. This gave the AOTA conference an aura of legitimacy and attracted physicians and other AHA members to AOTA events. Moreover, occupational therapists relied exclusively on physicians and AHA members for the leadership of the association from 1920 to 1938. During this period, the presidents of the AOTA included a physician interested in disability, an internationally known figure in rehabilitation, a psychiatrist who formerly chaired the New York State Hospital Commission, and a physician who earlier served as an AHA president.[76]

In short, occupational therapists surrendered leadership of their association to gain stature and increased use of their services. While they lost some control over the AOTA, the absence of subordinating ties to a medical specialty and the existence of a self-regulated mechanism restricting entry meant greater control over their own affairs following World War II. Thus organizational mechanisms developed for controlling entry would be less restrictive of their autonomy at a time when such autonomy became a goal of allied health occupations.

Again, this development arose less from planned action than from the market situation within which occupational therapists pursued their interests. Occupational therapists showed less political awareness at this time than did other groups. For example, physical therapy technicians had a standing legislative committee dating from the 1920s, while occupational therapists had none. Concern over licensing legislation did not appear until occupational therapists responded negatively to legislation passed for New York State nurses in 1938. Reacting to passage of remedial legislation to protect the public from unqualified nurses,[77] the association's journal reported that "registration was instituted by the A.O.T.A. to forestall such a step" and this registration "has heretofore been sufficient to keep out unqualified persons from practicing occupational therapy, but at almost any time some legislator may decide that members of the profession must have the endorsement of state authority in order to practice."[78] Indeed, the AOTA continued to resist licensing in favor of self-certification until the 1970s.

During the 1930s occupational therapy's isolation from other occupations began to change. Attempts by occupational therapists to widen the scope of their work led to conflicts with physical therapy technicians. Jurisdictional disputes occurred, especially in orthopedic and industrial accident cases, when occupational therapists staked a claim to exercise as a treatment for muscular and joint problems. Their expansion into the domain of physical therapy technicians was described by Kidner: "curative workshop has already, in many orthopedic hospitals, superseded the mechanotherapy room; with its elaborate equipment of mechanical apparatus for the correction of physical defect and the restoration of impaired muscular functions." This success, according to Kidner, was because patients preferred making something rather than doing passive exercise.[79]

"We are not trying to trespass on the physiotherapy field," claimed one occupational therapist trying to reduce tensions between the two groups, "we are simply dovetailing and supplementing and extending treatments by means of crafts."[80] Such "dovetailing" and "extending treatments" brought the work of occupational therapists into the physical therapy technicians' territory and forced clarification of the boundaries between them. Yet clarification was a difficult task because there was "no fine line of demarcation indicating where physiotherapy and occupational therapy begins and the other ends."[81] To distinguish their work from physical therapy, occupational therapists emphasized that they provided a more active treatment that involved the patient in psychologically meaningful activity, whereas the medical approach of physical therapy was more passive and narrower.[82] There was no attempt, however, to demarcate boundaries on the basis of specific body organs or types of disease. While it was agreed that occupational therapy usually followed physical therapy, there were no claims for the superiority of one method over the other in treating specific physical problems.[83]

Attempts by occupational therapists to define a unique place for themselves in hospitals created "complications and misunderstandings" with other occupations in the horizontal division of labor.[84] Tension between occupational therapists and social workers prompted one physician to write: "The idea of supremacy or that one department is arrogating, or trying to arrogate to itself undue credit or power should not exist and if it has arisen, it should be corrected."[85] The existence of a "cold and chilly atmosphere" and "uncomplimentary expressions and criticisms" between these departments must be replaced with a "close relationship" and "feeling of good-will."[86] A similar overlap in work fueled jealousies between occupational therapy and nursing. Therapists argued that nurses not only inappropriately provided occupational therapy to hospital patients without a physician's prescription[87] but also took credit for patients' recovery.[88] Even some hospital volunteers threatened occupational therapists when they were "over-zealous" and did "not discriminate who is 'boss.'"[89]

Growing concern was also shown by occupational therapists about their relationship to physical therapy physicians and their position in the vertical division of labor. Occupational therapists became increasingly wary of attempts by physical therapy physicians to define occupational therapy as a "highly specialized branch of physical therapy" to be closely supervised by a physical therapy physician.[90] There "seems to be an especial tendency," wrote one therapist, for members of the medical profession "to refuse to acknowledge occupational therapy as an entity, an adjunct to medical care and treatment, but to insist upon considering it as belonging to other therapeutic aids, such as physiotherapy."[91] Occupational therapists perceived such desires by physical therapy physicians as a threat to their goal for recognition as a distinct area of medical practice. While the physicians tried to assuage these fears by denying that occupational therapy departments in hospitals would become subordinate to physical therapy departments, physical therapy physicians were beginning to conceive of occupational therapy as lying in their domain and as subject to their authority.[92] The physicians, as part of their pursuit of specialty status and control of hospital physical therapy departments, sought to emphasize the close relationship between occupational and physical therapy to lay the foundation for eventual incorporation of occupational therapy.

Occupational therapists explored and expanded their relationship to physical therapy physicians, despite fears of losing autonomy and even occupational identity. In 1938 they accepted an invitation from the American Congress of Physical Therapy to hold their annual meetings jointly. "This event is highly significant," exclaimed the president of the AOTA, "and appears to indicate a closer relationship in the future between the practices of physical therapy and those of occupational therapy."[93] This acceptance broke the AOTA tradition of meeting with the AHA, and signaled a willingness to form closer ties with physical therapy physicians.[94]

Thus, the occupational therapists' position in the emerging division of labor was affected by factors that often operated at cross-purposes. One set of factors preserved some autonomy for occupational therapists: the variety of settings in which they practiced, their growing commitment to organizational devices that reinforced their professional identity, and their lack of competition with physical therapy physicians and others. This market situation and physical therapy physicians' focus on curative rather than rehabilitative medicine explains the disinterest of physicians in occupational therapy from 1920 to the mid-1930s. Also, the limited amount of competition from other groups meant less pressure for occupational therapists to establish protective alliances with medical specialties.

Another set of forces, which grew in significance during the late 1930s, reduced occupational therapy's autonomy. First, the concern over survival led to accrediting arrangements with the medical profession. Second, the prospect of war and the increased interest of physical therapy physicians provided a possibility for a stabler and more expanded role for occupational therapists. Although this resulted in a more subordinate relationship to physical therapy physicians, it greatly enhanced occupational therapy's position and ended its reliance on outside leadership after the war.

For physical therapy physicians, the new interest in occupational therapy was not due to the "natural" development of their methods in relation to rehabilitation, but to the AMA's recent change to tacit approval of specialization. Staking a claim to a unique territory was necessary to pursue specialty status. Although physical therapy physicians did not achieve formal specialty recognition and remained a marginal segment during the 1930s, they established the basis for eventual domination of the rehabilitation field. This domination was founded not only in their authority as physicians but also in their alliances with other groups. They assisted physical therapy technicians by arranging for the AMA to accredit technician schools. The existence of a similar mechanism for occupational therapists meant physical therapy physicians could indirectly control these two groups. More important, they achieved direct control over physical therapy technicians through the registry certifying entry into the occupation. Also, physical therapy physicians moved to increase their influence over occupational therapists by reestablishing contact toward the end of the 1930s. Unlike the situation in World War I, physical therapy physicians were prepared organizationally to respond to the opportunities of the forthcoming war.

5

The Rediscovery of
Rehabilitation, 1941–1950

Rehabilitation medicine's first fifty years had two phases. In the first and generally ignored phase, marginal medical practitioners organized around the use of electrical devices to treat acute diseases. The second phase covered the institutionalization of physical therapy from the beginning of World War I to the start of World War II. It included recognition by the military during the First World War, organization of a professional association by physical therapy physicians, and creation of physical and occupational therapy. It concluded with the physicians gaining control over the allied occupations and moving toward medical specialty status in the late 1930s. However, none of these developments occurred because of a gradual growth in the knowledge or technical base of the rehabilitation field; reconstruction and rehabilitation did not become an "emergent" core function for physical therapy physicians during the 1920s and 1930s.

Here we will describe a third phase in medical rehabilitation's history. If the first half-century of rehabilitation medicine was one of institutional change but therapeutic continuity, the 1940s brought institutional and therapeutic changes that culminated in specialty status. War again escalated the demand for medical services. For some physicians this resulted in a conflict between their imperialistic desires to control new opportunities and their tendency to resist increasing practitioner supply. This was not a problem for physical therapy physicians. An imperialistic posture had been their way of life for half a century, and practitioner shortage had been a crucial problem impeding their growth. They thus welcomed the chance to recruit new members and were relatively unconcerned about the lowering of standards in training programs.

While physical therapy physicians expanded their place in the military and the Veterans Administration (VA), they were not in the forefront of efforts to develop reconditioning and rehabilitation programs; innovation and program development came largely from those outside the physical therapy field. They did, however, incorporate new activities and alter their claims to expertise.

World War II and Physical Medicine

By the late 1930s physical therapy physicians were moving away from their original goal of becoming one part of a therapeutic triad for acute disease and toward the explicit pursuit of specialty status. Formal specialty recognition required physical therapy physicians to convince others that they possessed exclusive expertise over a specific set of medical problems or techniques. Although their position had improved, they still seemed a long way from establishing a claim to such special competence.

Krusen's "watermark" presidential address to the American Congress of Physical Therapy in 1938 delineated physical therapy's gains: "the medical profession has come to realize that not only chemicals, biologic preparations and surgical procedures, but also physical agents, may be of great value in combating disease, relieving suffering, and shortening disability."[1] However, he acknowledged the field's continued marginality: "As pioneers in a new field of medicine, we have had to contend with ultra-conservative physicians who doubted each of our forward steps. . . . A physician may inquire how many of the elaborate devices which we employ in physical therapy are discarded after a few months. He does not seem to realize that we strive to employ the simpler physical procedures whenever it is feasible."[2] His recommendations for increasing physical therapy's status in the medical profession included avoidance of the "spectacular," "half-truths," and "over-enthusiasm," as well as improvement of their own research and "condemnation of unscientific literature."[3]

Most notable was Krusen's unequivocal statement about the specialty status of physical therapy. He noted that "despite what anyone may say to the contrary . . . physical therapy is a specialty." However, he also claimed that the field should not be limited to physical therapy specialists, but that general practitioners should use simple physical therapies in their practices. "Just as the average physician may do his own urinalysis and blood counts but depends on the clinical pathologist for Wassermann reactions and blood chemical studies, so may he use an infra-red lamp or contrast baths in his own office. He may rely on the specialist in physical therapy for the more complicated procedures, such as fever therapy, or corrective exercises."[4]

In his speech, Krusen resurrected the strategy first enunciated in 1896 which sought to convince all to adopt physical therapy techniques while also claiming a special sphere of competence. This provided a way for a marginal group like physical therapy physicians to pursue control over a segment of the market without alienating the still powerful general practitioners on whom they depended for referrals. Such a strategy was ideologically safe because it did not claim that all physical therapy techniques required specialized competence. Given the jaundiced view of physical therapy still held by many physicians, such a claim would have met a great deal of resistance.

Physical therapy physicians developed a new conception of their mission as a response to organizational changes within the medical profession as well as in anticipation of war. As early as July 1938, an editorial linked physical therapy techniques to war needs; occupational therapy was specifically mentioned as an important facet of this work.[5] As the prospect of war heightened, the American Congress of Physical Therapy launched efforts to improve its position in the military. In June 1940 a letter to the surgeon general of the army offered assistance in setting up a physical therapy service in the army Medical Department.[6] One month later, an editorial entitled "Has the War Preparedness Committee Forgotten Physical Therapy?" underscored physical therapy's marginal position.[7] The editorial expressed "shock" over the omission of physical therapy from a questionnaire circulated by the AMA's War Preparedness Committee to provide manpower data to the army about physician availability. The editorial also stated that orthopedic surgeons' quasi-control over occupational therapy aides during World War I was due to a shortage of physical therapy physicians, implying that such work naturally fell within the purview of physical therapy. Underlying such editorializing was a fear that physical therapy physicians would again lose the war wounded to orthopedic departments, which were characterized as being staffed by "partially trained nurses, enlisted medical department personnel, or perchance young women who have taken a brief course in occupational therapy."

A later historical account singled out this strong editorial reaction as leading to "proper recognition being given the medical specialty by the Armed Services during World War II."[8] While this is an oversimplification, activities by the American Congress of Physical Therapy helped establish in 1942 a three-month program to train physicians in physical therapy techniques. During the war more than 300 physicians were trained in this program, thus preventing a shortage that would have given other groups a chance to extend their influence in the area.[9] The training of a large number of physicians in physical therapy techniques also helped the civilian situation after the war, since some of those trained remained in this field. As in World War I, this provided a favorable milieu for building occupational identities and a cadre of leaders who were able to maintain connections after the war.

The opportunity provided by war was crucial to physical

therapy physicians. Significantly, formal specialty status would be granted not in recognition of their traditionally claimed area of expertise, but for their capacity to shift the definition of their work to meet needs derived from war. This shift took the form, first evident in 1942, of claiming expertise in handling the convalescent phase of illness and the disabled in general. This focus on what was later to be termed the "third phase" of medicine was accompanied by a decline in claims to treat the acute phase of a wide variety of infirmities.

One event during this period, however, boosted the use of physical methods for acute care—the innovation in the treatment of poliomyelitis introduced to the United States in 1940 by Sister Kenny. Contrary to the traditional therapy, which called for immobility during the acute phase of illness, the Kenny method prescribed heat and motion. The *Archives of Physical Therapy* in January 1942 called this method "rather confused, probably due to lack of understanding of modern kinesiology."[10] Just five months later, however, Sister Kenny's praise was being sung in the following terms: "The medical profession owes a debt to Miss Kenny for her conception and for her vigorous support of her ideas."[11] In November, an entire issue of the *Archives* was devoted to her approach. This sudden change in attitude may have stemmed from the realization that this method could help advance physical therapy, especially since it argued against immobilizing measures frequently used by orthopedic surgeons. While focusing on acute care, the more activity-oriented therapy it prescribed was in line with increasing emphasis on patient activity, a change with which the physical therapy physicians would be intimately involved.

The idea of "total rehabilitation," dormant since World War I, was revived as a medical activity requiring special expertise. The physical therapy physicians also pushed a new concept of "prehabilitation" to transform an unfit civilian population into a fit military force.[12] This highly imperialistic conception held that physical therapy methods had utility to enhance and maintain health (prehabilitation), to treat acute injury and illness, and to rehabilitate convalescent patients.[13] While some, such as Krusen, hoped that physical therapy's involvement in prehabilitation work would extend to the civilian population, such a role never materialized, even in the military. In fact, no further mention of prehabilitation was made in the group's literature.

The Influence of "Outsiders"

Development of a connection between medicine and rehabilitation owed more to individuals outside physical therapy than to those within it. The internist Howard Rusk dates the beginning of medicine's interest in rehabilitation from his own work during World War II. He states, "Gradually the concept of rehabilitation came to me as I found out how much really could be done for these men." While self-serving, Rusk's version is accurate in tracing medicine's involvement with rehabilitation from the point where it "took off."[14]

Others have also claimed that their efforts were responsible for the development of medical involvement in physical medicine and rehabilitation. For example, Paul Magnuson, an orthopedic surgeon, states that the hospital department he organized and hired John Coulter to run "was the beginning of the science of physical medicine in this country." Coulter was one of the early leaders of physical therapy physicians and played a prominent role in the World War I military program.[15]

Yet Rusk, more than any other physician, is now associated with the beginning of the modern specialty of physical medicine. In 1942 he created a program in an air force hospital to make profitable use of convalescent time. He was soon brought to Washington to organize convalescent programs for the Army Air Force.[16] Initially, Rusk named the program the Army Air Force Reconditioning and Recreation Program, but he ran into immediate resistance from the Red Cross, which had legally defined rights to all recreation activities in the military. Rusk then stressed the program's training aspect and renamed it the Army Air Force Convalescent Training Program.

The Wadham Committee, appointed in 1942 to study military medical care, supported Rusk's desire for separate convalescent centers with a variety of services, but the surgeon general favored convalescent units in regular hospitals, apparently because he feared loss of control by the patient's original physician. In contrast to the surgeon general's position in World War I, the army wanted responsibility only for those returning to duty (reconditioning); those discharged would be the responsibility of the Veterans Administration (rehabilitation).[17] The White House presented a third plan, which would transfer responsibility for disabled veterans from the VA to the Office of Vocational Rehabilitation.[18] This position was consistent with White House desires during World War I to place responsibility with the civilian Federal Board of Vocational Education.

The struggle between these interests began with defeat of the LaFollette and Barden bill, which presented the White House plan. This bill was stiffly resisted by the VA and veterans' organizations as well as other groups who felt threatened, such as school superintendents and state interests representing the blind. A bill passed in March 1943 (P.L. 16) overcame the greatest source of resistance by providing for a totally independent veterans' program administered by the VA. Similarly, the complementary civilian bill, passed in July 1943 (P.L. 113), overcame resistance at the state level by placing control in the hands of state administrators and by providing separate programs for the blind.[19] By mid-1943, legislative steps had been taken to create a bureaucracy for rehabilitation of the war wounded and utilization of the civilian work force in a time of labor shortage.

The growth of the civilian rehabilitation program can be traced to this legislation. Particularly important was the 1943 Vocational Rehabilitation Law, which incorporated medical services. Although some physicians feared that this legislation was a cover for "socialized medicine," such resistance was overcome, thus opening the door for the expansion of physical medicine into civilian rehabilitation after the war.[20]

Those in vocational rehabilitation welcomed the inclusion of medical services that met a need and furthered their own occupational aspirations, previously stifled because of educator control over rehabilitation programs. The inclusion of medical services would allow them to dissociate from educational conceptions of their work, and to stress the individualized and therapeutic nature of their service. The creation of the Office of Vocational Rehabilitation in September 1943 was a symbol of, and a means for furthering, the separation of vocational rehabilitation from control by educators.[21]

In the military, Public Law 113 established a legal distinction, desired by both the army surgeon general and the VA, between "reconditioning" performed by the army and "rehabilitation" done by the VA. During the war, this distinction was never realized because the VA failed to develop adequate programs for dealing with the rehabilitation needs of those not returning to duty.[22] One observer of these events stated that the exact causes for VA failure will probably never be understood, but that they might lie with the conservatism of the VA leadership as well as with the conflicts between interested parties. In reference to the blinded soldier, this observer noted that the "extended haggling among the interested and the benevolent had resulted in the embarrassment of having a 'center for blinded veterans' approved by Congress, but never funded."[23]

The VA's failure provided Rusk and others with the opportunity to continue program development. This was so, even though they had no legal mandate to create such programs and they faced resistance from the army surgeon general, who had authority over the air force. Because VA programs were not organized until after the war, many of those involved in military rehabilitation would be instrumental in developing the VA approach to the disabled. This provided continuity between military and postwar VA programs.

During 1943 and most of 1944 the army and the air force continued to struggle over the nature of military rehabilitation. This resulted in a combination of different types of facilities that were underequipped and generally inadequate.[24] Meanwhile, Rusk continued to build his program by making important institutional connections, such as setting up a physician training program at the Institute for the Crippled and Disabled. He was also aided by personal connections to powerful individuals who could pressure for the extension of rehabilitation programs in the military. In particular, he gained the support of two persons close to the president, Eleanor Roosevelt and Bernard Baruch.

Baruch, whose father had been an early proponent of hydrotherapy, funded a committee in 1943 which would become an important mechanism in furthering the aspirations of physical therapy physicians. As a member of the Baruch Committee, Rusk prevailed on Baruch to go to the president and win his support for a military rehabilitation program. The White House initially favored civilian rehabilitation for those not returning to duty, but now backed Baruch's advocacy of military programs. The president's concurrence with Baruch's plan led to an order from the secretary of war that before discharge all military personnel should have "physical and psychological rehabilitation, vocational guidance, prevocational training and resocialization."[25] The surgeon general had been circumvented, and the necessary resources and authority were finally available to create rehabilitation programs during the last year of the war.

Expansion and a New Name

While these legislative and organizational developments were occurring between 1942 and 1944, the American Congress of Physical Therapy remained uninvolved politically. Instead, the physical therapy literature expressed general optimism over the spread of physical therapy techniques to other areas of medical practice and pushed for recognition of physical therapy physician expertise in a wider scope of medical work.[26] Given their continued marginal position, the focus by physical therapy physicians on these limited goals is not surprising; they lacked the power to make an impact on larger issues. Although they expressed interest in increasing their involvement in rehabilitation, they had not yet tied their fortunes to the handling of convalescent patients. Not until 1945, when the military rehabilitation program rapidly expanded, did rehabilitation become central to their interests.

A 1941 editorial in the *Archives of Physical Therapy* articulated the requirements for future development of the field: foundation support, increased attention to research, and the founding of a "great" institute of physical medicine at a university.[27] One year later, the presidential address at the annual conference sounded a similar theme, calling for both basic and clinical research and stating that physical medicine was staging an "invasion" of the specialties: "For many years physical medicine has been the handmaiden of orthopedics, but now we see its increasing use in neurology and psychiatry, in dermatology, in internal medicine, in pediatrics, in urology, in surgery, in otolaryngology, and even in ophthalmology." The author tied further expansion to dissemination of knowledge about the physiologic effects of their techniques.[28]

Formation of the Baruch Committee on Physical Medicine proved critical to the realization of their goals. The committee sought to improve physical medicine's scientific basis and to push for its recognition by the medical community. The committee's first report, published in early 1944, stated that "the last war is said to have established orthopedic surgery as a recognized specialty [and that] this war may do the same for physical medicine."[29] Committee members lauded the field's wide scope: "This extensive field of medical practice includes the employment of the physical and other effective properties of light, heat, cold, water, electricity, massage, manipulation, exercise, and mechanical devices for physical and occupational therapy, in the diagnosis and treatment of disease." Physical medicine was also portrayed as a preventive measure for certain diseases, such as joint and muscle problems, and its use was recommended for industrial medicine, geriatrics, and the treatment of rheumatic diseases and diseases of the blood vessels and nervous system.[30]

The committee identified three major needs facing physical medicine. First, an "adequate supply" of physical therapy physicians was needed. The committee recommended establishing fellowships, creating a "circuit rider" to consult with schools in setting up programs, and launching a public relations program to promote "proper recognition" of the field through "discriminating publicity."[31] The second need was to advance the status of the field by increasing basic and clinical research.[32] This research was to be rooted in biophysics, thereby providing the scientific basis for the segment's diagnostic and therapeutic techniques.[33] Third, the committee addressed use of physical medicine in the war and provided links to the postwar civilian situation.[34] One military physician, in a letter to the committee, noted that "if rehabilitation in the armed forces is under the direction of medical officers, as it certainly should be, the medical profession now in civilian life will profit by example and upon demobilization a number of men trained by experience in these procedures will be returned to civil life and may be expected to continue."[35]

The Baruch Committee still considered rehabilitation as one area of practice among many in physical medicine, but others disagreed. Most extreme were people like Rusk, who believed that rehabilitation should constitute a separate specialty field. Another school of thought held that rehabilitation should become the purview of those in physical medicine who had the necessary expertise for supervising such work. A third group argued that rehabilitation should be part of all medical practice rather than the prerogative of one specialty. Whatever their disagreements, the major interested parties all agreed with the Baruch Committee's position that medical supervision of rehabilitation "cannot be dispensed with except at the greatest risk. Rehabilitation must remain firmly under medical control."[36]

One year later the Baruch Committee reported its accomplishments. A central office to serve as a clearinghouse and disburser of grants had been created, model projects at Columbia, New York University, and the Medical College of Virginia had been supported, and research and teaching at other medical schools had been funded. The committee also pointed to the successful transfer of physical and occupational therapy from Columbia Teachers' College to the physical medicine department of its medical school at Bellevue Hospital.[37] Similarly, assistance from the Baruch Committee helped reorganize the University of Illinois College of Medicine to form a new Department of Physical Medicine with authority over physical and occupational therapy.[38]

The Baruch Committee had become a symbol of physical medicine's increased importance and a powerful mechanism for furthering this group's position and interests. As a long-time leader in the field recently commented, the committee served to "infuse with new life and strength and vigor a struggling and heretofore discouraged field of medicine."[39] It accomplished this by funding activities such as research and public relations. The committee also provided political power by legitimating physical therapy physicians' work and by affording access, through Bernard Baruch, to persons of power. Institutional structures created by the Baruch Committee made possible continued efforts to gain acceptance and to expand in the postwar years.

These institutional improvements lent support to the broadening conception of physical medicine practice to include reconditioning and rehabilitation through "scientific" diagnosis and treatment. The case for reconditioning as the "scientific organization of convalescence" (as distinct from the restoration of earning power in "rehabilitation") was made in the *Archives* in 1945: the wartime experience showed that "the main features of a well-organized reconditioning program would automatically fall into the enlarged scope of the departments of physical medicine."[40] In staking claims to the management of convalescence it was necessary to attack previous reliance on rest as the prescribed treatment during the convalescent phase. These attacks began at war's end. One author asserted that the virtue of rest as a therapeutic procedure had been extolled so long that it was "almost considered heresy to describe any deleterious effects which could be directly attributed to this general procedure."[41] As another author pointed out, however, the use of activity was not really new; there had been physicians recommending early mobilization and activity after surgery since 1899.[42]

In the words of the Baruch Committee, physical medicine would take up "the dead space between definitive care and ability to return to productive work, the setup for retraining and reconditioning, medicine and its relation to environment, occupation, social status, etc." Physical medicine was a "new concept as far as the general medical profession is concerned."[43] The committee also stated that the entire medical profession saw "the necessity of reorienting much of their knowledge to the demands of a broadening social conception of medicine. The horizons of mental and physical health are extending to areas hitherto regarded as belonging exclusively to other professions."[44]

The improving situation for physical therapy physicians was also reflected in internal developments during this period. Reconceptualization of their domain led them to consider a new name for their field. One *Archives* editorial suggested that physical therapy physicians rename their specialty "external" or "parietal medicine," "rehabilitation," or "physical medicine."[45] The editorial was followed by a letter from a physician who recommended the name "physicology" because this term showed the connection between physics and physiology.[46] Subsequently, others recommended titles such as "physiomedy" and "physiatry."[47]

In 1944, their name was changed to physical medicine through a resolution at the annual meeting of the American Congress of Physical Therapy.[48] The field's new name was heralded as emphasizing the "scientific and diagnostic basis of the medical use of physical agents" rather than "the purely clinical." Moreover, the new name was thought to "lend more dignity to its practitioners" and to help "overcome much of the confusion by the indiscriminate use of the term 'physical therapist' by both physicians and technicians."[49] Legitimation of their diagnostic skill strengthened their claim to a scientific basis in "medical physics"[50] and their position within the patient care hierarchy. In short, the aspiring specialty would find it increasingly intolerable to follow the instructions of primary care physicians.

Physical medicine physicians then turned to what they should call themselves. After two years of deliberation, members of the American Congress of Physical Medicine chose "physiatrist," a combination of the Greek *physis* (nature) and *iatreia* (healing). Although they admitted this designation would "sound strange when first used," it was believed "that the medical profession as well as the public will become used to it."[51] This title, still in use today, was officially adopted in 1946 after approval by the AMA's Council on Physical Medicine.

Finally, the Baruch Committee and the Council on Physical Medicine began to push for specialty recognition by requesting a permanent section in the AMA from the Council on Scientific Assembly, and by forming the American Board of Physical Medicine to handle certification.[52] These efforts reached culmination in 1947 when the American Board of Physical Medicine gave its first examination.[53]

By 1947 physiatrists achieved AMA specialty recognition. They succeeded in parlaying war opportunities into formal specialty status with claimed expertise in the diagnostic and therapeutic use of physical agents and in the supervision and coordination of allied health workers. They also altered their focus from acute care to the treatment of convalescent and chronic problems. At the same time, they were beginning to articulate a therapeutic regimen based on activity and exercise rather than inactivity and rest.

Allied Occupations in the War

Physical Therapy

Physical therapy technicians struggled between the wars to acquire military status equivalent to the Army Nurses Corps. They increased training from four months to a full year, and by the late 1930s also required prospective trainees to have a bachelor's degree in physical education. Originally short courses had been accepted, but this stopped in order to recruit persons with a "physical therapy viewpoint."[54] At the brink of World War II, physical therapy technicians still had not gained military status, although they had achieved civil service recognition. Because of their nonprofessional status in the Civil Service Commission, however, the Commission retained power to set standards for allied health personnel. Especially noxious to the allied occupations was the Commission's policy of meeting personnel needs by substituting experience for educational requirements.[55]

When the war began, technicians worried about competition from "advertising commercial schools which adhere to no particular standards [and] are turning out each year large numbers of inadequately prepared technicians . . . [while] there is an acute shortage of graduates of approved schools."[56] American Physiotherapy Association (APA) concern was "over the contingency of lowered standards should the demand [for physical therapy technicians] exceed the supply."[57]

To meet demand, the APA and the AMA's Council on Physical Therapy and Council on Medical Education and Hospitals jointly established accelerated courses that produced technicians with a civil service rating of "apprentice physiotherapy aide." The only difference between these aides and fully qualified technicians was that they had less clinical practice. The emphasis was on maintaining the highest possible standards by distinguishing newer trainees from those who met the higher prewar civilian requirements. An editorial in the *Physiotherapy Review* reflected the sanctity of these standards: "The present high standards of education did not just happen. Today they are taken for granted but many of us remember the long struggle to raise those standards."[58] In agreements made with both AMA councils it was understood that they would revert to their original standards after the war.

The APA had former and inactive members take the place of the civilians going into service "to protect the home field from pseudotherapists who might take advantage of the emergency." This fear of losing out to civilian competitors was not seen as a "race" to siphon students away from the military but as "an earnest desire on the part of all concerned to be able to administer physical therapy to all who needed it."[59] A proposal to increase the number of technicians through War Department subsidies to civilian schools was rejected by the surgeon general.[60]

In 1940 the APA formed a Relations Committee to improve connections with affiliated local societies and to place APA representatives on committees and programs of related organizations. Through its efforts the APA was represented in the American Association for Health, Physical Education and

Recreation; Advisory Committee of the National Foundation for Infantile Paralysis; Subcommittee on Clinical Research of the Baruch Committee; Advisory Board, Federal Security Agency, Rehabilitation Division; and the National Council on Rehabilitation (which the APA helped found in 1942). In addition, the APA received grants from the Kellogg and Rosenberg foundations as well as the Baruch Committee and the National Foundation for Infantile Paralysis. Some of these grants were specifically for the purpose of "advancing the general cause of physical therapy" by adding staff to the APA and through publicity.[61]

This new communications network allowed the APA to pressure congressmen for improvements in the military status of physical therapy technicians. The APA suggested that members write to congressmen emphasizing the length of their training, the high standards of their association, and their cooperation with the AMA over these standards.[62] Thus, on the basis of their standards and their relationship to the AMA, technicians claimed full military status under the surgeon general rather than the Civil Service Commission.

Legislation granting technicians "relative rank" was passed in 1942. Two years later they gained commissioned officer status and apprentice physiotherapy aides became noncommissioned officers. Such military adoption of existing specialty designations served to formalize emerging occupational boundaries.[63] Issuing new uniforms and dropping the term "aide" constituted important symbolic changes. Physician adoption of the term "physical medicine"[64] left allied workers free to call themselves physical therapists. As regular military personnel, physical therapists were removed from Civil Service Commission regulation and placed under the surgeon general's control. Civilian physical therapists remained under Civil Service control until after the war.[65]

The changed locus of control was important because the surgeon general protected allied occupations from Civil Service Commission attempts to override educational requirements. The commission could still avoid such requirements by invoking the Veterans' Preference Act of 1944, which made it possible for them to be waived for veterans in "nonprofessional" fields. In one instance the commission sought to overcome educational requirements for dietitians, but the surgeon general protested and the commission dropped the matter.[66]

Procurement of physical therapists, formerly the duty of the Civil Service Commission and the Red Cross, became the responsibility of the more effective Officer Procurement Service of the Army in 1943. The service's nationwide publicity network reached high schools and colleges and "people throughout the country were made aware of the term 'physical therapist.'"[67] In all, slightly more than half of the 1,600 physical therapists produced during the war received their training in military programs.[68]

Despite these changes in status, numbers, and public awareness, physical therapy remained subservient to medicine. As noted above, physical therapists worked closely with the AMA Council on Medical Education and Hospitals to win approval of wartime training programs and to preserve their standards. The medical profession extended its control over physical therapy in 1945 through the addition of a requirement in the council's "Essentials of an Acceptable School for Physical Therapy Technicians" which required physical therapists to work under physician direction.[69] For the most part, physical therapists did not oppose this relationship with physicians.

Years earlier the New York Medical Practice Act (of 1926) granted physical therapists a license to practice in their own offices if supervised by a physician. By 1943, "licensed physical therapists" not affiliated with the APA supported a New York bill permitting practice without any medical supervision. But, anxious to remain under the medical profession's protective umbrella, the APA affiliate in New York joined with the profession to defeat this bill.[70] Here, and in a similar situation in Maryland, the APA advised its local affiliates to work with physical therapy's "best ally," the medical societies.[71]

The physical medicine segment was especially concerned about this attempt to "practice medicine": "the medical profession was put to endless waste of time and energy to defeat this demand, which is of course both unwarranted and dangerous from the standpoint of public health." Those physical therapy technicians aligned with the medical profession depended on the "good will of the medical profession [rather than] being involved in time wasting and essentially futile efforts for legislative wire-pulling." The American Registry of Physical Therapy Technicians, run by the American Congress of Physical Therapy, was pointed to as providing national standards to overcome problems resulting from "legislative zeal" in some states.[72]

In its internal communications the APA referred to the actions of these licensed physical therapists as its "union problem" in New York. The issue of licensing was raised at the 1944 national meeting but was little discussed, and no decision was reached.[73] Evidently, interest in gaining autonomy depended on local situations; the New York effort did not represent a major thrust to become independent from the medical profession. The issue of legislation to license physical therapy technicians was to grow in significance after the war.

Conflicts with other groups occasionally arose within military reconditioning and rehabilitation programs. One conflict occurred among physical therapists, occupational therapists, and prosthetists over amputee cases. The surgeon general resolved the conflict by giving physical therapy a mandate to handle the patient prior to fitting of the prosthesis. After fitting, those with upper extremity amputations were to be handled by occupational therapy and those with lower extremity amputations by physical therapy.[74] After the prosthetist had brought the prosthesis to the physical therapy department, the actual fitting of the lower extremity prosthesis was to be done in the presence of the physical therapist.

Occupational therapists, however, desired a greater role with lower extremity cases as these accounted for eighty percent of all amputations. While admitting that their work with these cases was primarily "diversional," occupational therapists wished to play a "supplementary" role to physical therapy in teaching patients to use prostheses and in prevocational training.[75] The division of labor based on upper and lower extremities was maintained, however, and was also followed in the VA as well as in many civilian institutions. At present it is less important than it was in the early postwar period.[76]

As physical therapy's connection with the medical profession tightened so did its connection with physical medicine. The latter relationship became increasingly desirable for both groups; it helped physical medicine to solidify control over its expanding "empire" and physical therapy to improve its commodity status and the demand for service. These interests converged in 1946, when physical therapy, occupational therapy, and physical reconditioning were placed under the army's new Physical Medicine Consultants' Division.[77]

After the war physical therapists strengthened control over a piece of the medical market and improved their professional stature. They were especially concerned with the nonprofessional ranking given physical therapists in the Civil Service Commission which allowed the commission to circumvent APA educational requirements. Standards lowered during the war were increased to distinguish themselves further from nursing and physical education. They even considered establishing a four-year physical therapy education program.[78] In addition to seeking government subsidization of demand for rehabilitation services, the APA wanted to influence state and national planning for rehabilitation and more generally demonstrate the value of their cause and organization. These goals were pursued by closely following legislative developments at the local and national levels.[79]

Occupational Therapy

Although occupational therapy had begun a rapprochement with the medical profession by the late 1930s, the period between the wars had been difficult for them. In the military, they pressed for longer training programs and in 1924 won approval of a six-month program. This was extended to nine months in 1932, although a request for an eleven-month course was rejected. In 1933 the military stopped training occupational therapists, physical therapists, and dietitians. Although training for the latter two groups soon resumed, this was not the case for occupational therapists. By 1939 there were fewer than a dozen occupational therapists on duty in the military.[80]

While physical therapy technicians and dietitians were granted military status and placed directly under medical supervision, occupational therapists continued as part of the Civil Service Commission. The surgeon general continued to view occupational therapy as a diversional activity rather than as a medically "essential" acute-care service.[81] In the therapists' view, failure to gain military status was undesirable because the commission ignored educational requirements in meeting manpower needs.[82]

AOTA began its campaign for military status by forming the Committee on Occupational Therapy and National Defense, and the War Service Committee.[83] At the same time, the Public Education Committee embarked on a "nationwide drive" to publicize occupational therapy and to demonstrate its value as a "medical treatment."[84] These committees recommended that physicians supervise occupational therapists with separate sections for neuropsychiatric and orthopedic work, and that occupational therapists supervise Red Cross and recreational workers.[85]

Recommending these separate sections indicates that occupational therapists did not yet conceive of their position in the medical division of labor as falling under the authority of physical medicine, which was still viewed as part of orthopedic work. These recommendations also revealed occupational therapy's concern over the use of volunteers and recreation workers, whose work was labeled "diversional" as opposed to "therapeutic." Especially problematic was the absence of regular occupational therapists in the war zone. Instead, programs run by volunteers or enlisted people skilled in a trade were often called "occupational therapy." Others were headed by a nurse and could not so easily be discounted; these were criticized as paying insufficient attention to the individual patient's situation.[86]

To carry out the recommendations the AOTA exerted pressure at the state and national levels and enlisted the aid of sympathetic physicians, some of whom were AOTA leaders. As a result, occupational therapists were offered commissions in the Women's Army Corps, but they rejected this proposal.[87] What they wanted were commissions in the military's medical program similar to those granted to dietitians and physical therapists.

A major improvement in occupational therapy's situation occurred when the National Research Council's Division of

Medical Sciences created a Conference on Occupational Therapy to push for military status under medical supervision. The AOTA's War Service Committee placed a representative on this Conference and became involved with joint meetings of the Conference, Medical Corps of the War Department, and Civil Service Commission. One aim of the War Service Committee and the Conference on Occupational Therapy was to change occupational therapy's civil service classification from "Trades and Industries" to "Medical Division."[88]

While they remained under the authority of the Civil Service Commission, the military Medical Department countered the threat to occupational therapy's "professional" standards. The surgeon general "assisted" in the procurement of occupational therapists, required professional education consistent with AOTA standards, and rejected as "unqualified" those therapists sent by the commission. When the last tactic failed, the individual was often disqualified later for not meeting physical or academic standards.[89] Thus, the Civil Service Commission's authority over acquisition and deployment of occupational therapists was undermined by the surgeon general, who acted to preserve his own authority over all aspects of the military medical effort.

Organizationally, occupational therapists were under the authority of either orthopedic surgery or neuropsychiatry. In 1943 they were transferred to the newly constituted Reconditioning Division, headed by a physician friendly to occupational therapy, where they remained for the duration of the war.[90] Having a sympathetic division head was important because appointments of occupational therapists were restricted to graduates of accredited schools or to those registered with the AOTA.

In mid-1944 the War Department finally initiated an emergency war course to train occupational therapists. This was a significant development, as a symbol of military medical recognition and for the increase of the supply of therapists.[91] By the end of the war there were 447 graduate occupational therapists and 452 apprentices working in the military medical system.[92]

By again stressing the therapeutic nature of their work, occupational therapists moved more securely under medical protection and domination. More significant, the rediscovery of rehabilitation made the medical profession more aware of occupational therapy because of its potential to bridge the physical and vocational aspects of rehabilitation.

Physical medicine physicians were especially interested in broadening the role of occupational therapy. The *Report of the Baruch Committee on Physical Medicine* attributed occupational therapy's lack of growth to its "sterile preoccupation" with "arty" pursuits such as basketry and weaving. It stated that "occupational therapy has been covering only a limited portion of its proper field . . . and that it should have more contact with medicine . . . where it rightfully belonged."[93] Moving to consolidate and extend their gains, physical medicine physicians now saw occupational therapy "as a phase of physical medicine" rather than as part of neuropsychiatry or orthopedics.[94]

Most occupational therapists welcomed adoption of the medical model and increased subservience to medicine. However, a few questioned the closer relationship with physical medicine and argued for continued contact with primary physicians of all specialty backgrounds. In the years to come occupational therapists increasingly saw little benefit in their closer association with physical medicine. Instead, therapists began to see this relationship as a vehicle for the promotion of physical medicine's empire.[95]

Occupational therapists also faced boundary disputes with other groups as their involvement deepened with medicine and rehabilitation. The potential for conflict increased as occupational therapists assumed new responsibilities. Some of these tasks included prosthetic training, making orthotic devices, training in activities of daily living, progressive restive exercises, vocational evaluation and training, therapeutic use of self, working with unconscious needs, using groups, and formulating psychodynamics on the basis of patients' artwork.[96] Potential conflict existed, then, with virtually every group in the modern rehabilitation division of labor, including orthotics-prosthetics, corrective therapy, rehabilitation counseling, art therapy, and social work.

In the 1940s, actual problems did exist among occupational therapy, physical therapy, and vocational rehabilitation. These struggles were reflected in calls for intergroup coordination and conflict resolution in individual work situations.[97] In short, occupational therapy had become part of the expanding and increasingly complex division of labor in rehabilitation.

Early Postwar Years

Immediately following the war, physical medicine's domain reached its height through reorganization of the military medical department and dissemination of ideas and programs created in the military to other institutions, most notably the Veterans Administration. Physical medicine finally acquired control over military rehabilitation when the army established the Physical Medicine Consultants' Division in 1946. Physical therapy, an enlarged occupational therapy, and physical reconditioning services were placed under the direction of physical medicine.[98] This reorganization initially applied to hospitals with more than 750 beds. For smaller hospitals, physical therapy remained under the Orthopedic Section, and occupational therapy and reconditioning under the Reconditioning Division. Also, a Convalescent Services Division was organized to handle the "nonprofessional functions" (e.g., recreation and education). In the process, physical therapists heading hospital departments were replaced by physiatrists.[99] Displacement was especially difficult for physical therapists, who were accustomed to relating directly to chiefs of other hospital services and to participating in hospital staff conferences.

In general, both physical therapy and occupational therapy lost some control over their own administrative and professional affairs. Physiatrists could now screen referrals from other physicians and prescribe physical and occupational therapy to patients.[100] This arrangement was praised at the time as one to be emulated in the civilian sphere: "Civilian hospitals should follow in the lead of military hospitals in better coordination of Physical Therapy, Occupational Therapy, and rehabilitation under the direction of a qualified medical specialist in Physical Medicine."[101] This extension of physical medicine created a current of dissatisfaction among displaced physical therapists,[102] and, at a more general level, a negative reaction among the growing allied occupations. As their status and security improved, the allied occupations increasingly resisted physical medicine's control over their work and professional activities.

The Veterans Administration

Medical rehabilitation's development in the VA after the war had significant impact on the future division of labor. The VA medical program in the 1940s has been called the "golden days"[103] of the VA's Medical Department, as well as a time of "building an empire."[104] This was especially true for the rehabilitation program, and specifically for physical medicine. At various times over the next two decades, the Physical Medicine and Rehabilitation Division of the VA included the following groups: physical therapy, occupational therapy, corrective therapy, manual arts therapy, industrial therapy, education therapy, recreation therapy, speech and hearing, and blind rehabilitation. Their struggles with one another, as well as with physiatrists and the VA medical hierarchy, began shortly after the war and continue today.

War-related demand for medical and rehabilitative services prompted legislative and administrative actions to reorganize the VA. These actions turned the VA into an arena for empire building. At the end of the war, General Omar Bradley was named to head the VA, and General Paul Hawley, who served in the war with Bradley, became the chief medical director. They obtained congressional authorization to establish a new VA department of medicine and surgery and embarked on "General Bradley's cleanup."[105] Interestingly, Bernard Baruch was a friend of Bradley's. While developing plans for the VA medical program, Bradley reportedly contacted Baruch and relied on the reports of the Baruch Committee on Physical Medicine.[106]

Paul Magnuson, an orthopedic surgeon who later succeeded Hawley, organized the "Deans Committee System" to connect VA hospitals with local medical schools. The "system" provided a means for tapping medical school faculties, and especially for enlisting the help of physicians who were instrumental in the military medical program. In this way, Donald Covalt was brought in to head the physical medicine and rehabilitation department, while Rusk and Krusen served as program consultants.

In his autobiography Rusk stated that he was asked by President Truman to help reorganize the VA programs. To this end, he attended a Potsdam conference in the guise of serving as personal physician to one of the participants in order to influence Bradley, who was to take over the VA.[107] While Rusk was a consultant in medical rehabilitation, Krusen consulted in physical medicine. Krusen embraced the new work in rehabilitation as a natural part of physical medicine, but he maintained that physical medicine should be the core task of the specialty.[108]

The Civil Service Commission's authority to determine personnel policies prevented these physicians from re-creating and extending programs that existed in the military. With the support of powerful veterans' groups, however, the VA medical department lobbied successfully for Public Law 293, which ended commission authority.[109] This law opened the way for physicians in physical medicine to create and control a division of labor.

Of course they still faced constraints in pursuing these goals. Ongoing conflicts occurred between the department of medicine and surgery and the vocational rehabilitation and education program. The head of the latter reportedly resisted sharing rehabilitation tasks with the former.[110] Also, General Carl Gray, who succeeded Bradley, sought to increase administrative prerogatives at the expense of the professional control desired by the chief medical director, Magnuson. Gray attempted to lessen the authority of the medical profession in the VA; the consequent struggle resulted in a congressional subcommittee hearing, which recommended medical control. Magnuson responded, "in the V.A., the doctor is master in his own house."[111]

The Physical Medicine and Rehabilitation Service

Implementation of the concept of a "third phase" of medicine called "medical rehabilitation" first occurred in the VA. Reportedly, fear existed in some medical circles that "medical rehabilitation" implied a movement toward socialized medicine, and thus the service was eventually named "Physical Medicine and Rehabilitation."[112] The medical rehabilitation service was originally organized into several sections including physical medicine, industrial therapy, aural rehabilitation, and rehabilitation of the blind.[113] This arrangement placed physical medicine in direct control of physical and occupational therapy and the new field of corrective physical training, later known as corrective therapy.

At first, medical rehabilitation was organizationally separate from industrial therapy, but redefinition of education and shop retraining work as a form of medical therapy gave rise to the fields of educational therapy and manual arts therapy. Their primary responsibility was to provide treatment, and secondarily to impart knowledge and skill. Although a lay executive officer was responsible for nonmedical supervision, the work of these occupations was to be prescribed by a physiatrist.[114] Physical medicine's authority over the two groups had been ambiguous until their work was redefined as therapeutic and included in the VA's expanding medical sphere under the supervision of physicians. Many years later this foray into educational and vocational work was justified in the following terms: "Because the V.A. was responsible for the medical well-being and the vocational future of discharged servicemen, it was necessary to extend services available under medical direction to encompass educational and vocational activities."[115]

Even more ambiguous was the relationship between physical medicine and those fields that worked with the vision, hearing, or speech impaired. Programs serving the blind have typically enjoyed a degree of autonomy. State commissions for the blind, for example, are frequently separate from other vocational rehabilitation units. Such relative autonomy within the VA medical system has been the result of an organized power base rather than an occupational strength.

The major group working with the blind, today known as "orientation and mobility instructors," was created in the VA. Those who struggled to build a program for the blind tried to develop a VA staff completely responsible for rehabilitation and free from the authority of other units. Existing allied occupations in the Physical Medicine and Rehabilitation Service, however, resisted the development of a new occupation. The strongest opposition came from corrective therapy, which "looked on it as something which belonged in the province they were developing." Once resistance was overcome, the chief of corrective therapy loaned some of his own therapists to become the nucleus of the orientation and mobility instructors. These instructors organized and grew within the VA, and eventually spread to civilian practice in the 1950s.[116]

In the 1950s, conferences whose participants included government, private groups, foundations, and leaders of the orientation and mobility instructors were held to discuss future development. It was decided that mobility instructors should have at least one year of graduate training; this was supported by the Office of Vocational Rehabilitation. Civilian development of the field was largely dependent on government financial support, although it is reported that the mobility people are now "on their own." At present, a master's degree is required and attempts to gain state licensing legislation have been made.[117] In the VA, they have maintained their autonomy vis-à-vis physical medicine physicians. While sometimes falling under the authority of physical medicine in specific hospitals, the mobility instructors are free from control by physical medicine in the central office in Washington, D.C.

Those dealing with speech and hearing problems have also maintained a greater degree of autonomy than other groups. In this case, occupational group strength was a significant factor. As one observer noted, the speech people, being mainly

Ph.D.s, did not belong under physical medicine, but there was "no place else to put them."[118] In the VA, speech pathologists were placed in the Physical Medicine and Rehabilitation Service until 1965, but were not required to work under the direct supervision of physicians. Physical medicine physicians unsuccessfully sought to prescribe the work of speech therapists and to create a registry similar to that for physical therapists. The speech therapists have remained free of control by physical medicine, both in the VA and in the civilian sphere.

Again, speech pathologists in the VA may be placed in hospital physical medicine and rehabilitation departments, but they remain outside physical medicine's authority in the central office. In civilian hospitals they may also be in physical medicine and rehabilitation but are likely to retain considerable autonomy. For example, at Montefiore Hospital in New York, the Speech and Hearing unit is under medical rehabilitation; all patients are first seen by a physiatrist, who can request an evaluation but cannot prescribe a particular speech therapy service.[119]

Physical medicine moved to strengthen control over speech and hearing workers in the 1960s. Reflecting these workers' lack of interest in a closer alliance with physical medicine, the American Speech and Hearing Association (ASHA) appealed in 1961 to the National Commission on Accreditation (NCA) to become the accrediting body for training programs. The NCA sought the opinion of the AMA, which argued against such approval on the grounds that it was unclear where the "medical direction lies." Instead, the AMA envisioned a collaborative program and, interestingly, mentioned psychiatry and EENT, but not physical medicine, as potential collaborators. Denying it was empire building, the AMA stated that its concerns derived from the close relationship between the fields and the desire to avoid "unpleasant situations," as had occurred with nursing, for example.[120]

ASHA replied that its members constituted a unique discipline, different from "paramedical technicians," and that their work was "psycho-educational," involving the development of communication skills and not the provision of medical treatment.[121] They complained of a "major misunderstanding" with physical medicine, which was seen as claiming speech therapy without thoroughly understanding the field. Speech pathologists did not attempt to define their work as medical treatment to the degree that other allied occupations had. Having spun off from the National Association of Teachers of Speech during the 1920s and 1930s, they sought acceptance from the medical profession but never rejected their educational roots. Their efforts to gain approval from the medical profession included reliance on physician leadership of their association during the late 1930s and articles calling for closer cooperation between speech pathology and medicine.[122]

Physical medicine continued to stake a claim over speech pathology. A 1972 report on medical rehabilitation in the VA stated that speech therapy was "an integral part" of medical rehabilitation. The report noted "a basic similarity between the re-education of the speech musculature as done by the speech therapist and the re-education of other body muscles as done by the physical therapist." In conclusion, the report said that the total medical rehabilitation program should "be under unified medical direction which is presently lacking in speech therapy."[123]

After several meetings, ASHA agreed to include two representatives from the AMA's Council on Medical Education and Hospitals on the accrediting body to formulate and implement requirements for training institutions. It also agreed that a physician would go on all site visits.[124] ASHA thus avoided efforts by physical medicine and rehabilitation to reassert and extend control over speech pathology, but accepted AMA participation in its accreditation activities to gain NCA recognition. In short, ASHA created a basis for partial autonomy.

The Allied Occupations

The struggles among allied therapy groups over a place in the division of labor were more problematic than their relationship to physical medicine. Physical medicine's claim to coordination of the rehabilitation team and scientific management of convalescence was based on its authority over allied occupations. Conflict among these occupations jeopardized physical medicine's claim to head the rehabilitation team.

The major overlap occurred between physical therapy and corrective therapy, and between occupational therapy and both manual arts therapy and educational therapy. The first attempt to coordinate these groups came in 1949, when the Central Medical Division ordered the consolidation of educational therapy and manual arts therapy with occupational therapy. Confronted by great resistance, this directive was eventually rescinded in 1952.[125] Interlocking occupational interests in the Physical Medicine and Rehabilitation Service blocked reorganization because it threatened survival of these two occupations.

A more direct conflict, with important implications for the civilian sphere, occurred between physical therapy and corrective therapy. Corrective therapists got their start during the war because of the shortage of physical therapists.[126] Initially, physical educators were recruited and trained to provide "exercise therapy" for psychiatric patients in the military. Later, they worked with the war wounded and were brought to the VA by physicians, like Rusk, who used them during the war.[127]

The fact that corrective therapists were men and physical therapists were almost all women affected this conflict. The military and VA preferred to have men handle physical exercise, which became the core task of corrective therapists (reconditioning work directed by women may have run counter to prevailing sex role stereotypes). Ideological attacks launched by corrective therapy argued that female physical therapists were not strong enough to deal with paraplegics.[128]

The only conflict between physical therapy and corrective therapy in the wartime army involved a dispute over the amputee walking program. A directive from the surgeon general gave full responsibility to physical therapists.[129] However, placing these two groups together in the VA quickly produced a heated struggle. To distinguish their work, physical therapy focused on the injured part of the body and corrective therapy the noninjured part (one was passive, the other active).[130] This distinction did little to allay the problem. Physical therapy charged that corrective therapy uselessly duplicated its own functions, while corrective therapy fought for a place in the rehabilitation division of labor.

Although some physical medicine physicians in the VA supported corrective therapists, the American Congress of Physical Medicine argued that the civilian sector had no need for an occupation so similar to physical therapy. An *Archives* editorial stated that "physical therapy by a simple process of expansion in training and practice could adequately assume the bulk of the work which is now being done by corrective physical rehabilitation [corrective therapy]."[131] But physical therapy was unwilling to alter its focus, as was shown by the neglect of "therapeutic exercise" in its teaching and practice.

Physical medicine resisted corrective therapy's extension to the civilian sphere because it had an existing relationship and commitment to physical therapy and was concerned over corrective therapists' lack of medical knowledge. Physiatrists pointed to their long involvement with physical therapy in raising the group's standards, and claimed that inclusion of corrective therapists in civilian practice posed a threat to these standards.[132] Moreover, in the civilian sphere physiatrists had less control over corrective therapists. In terms of potential economic competition and coordination of a division of labor, physiatrists would have had to assist the professionalization of corrective therapists and develop mechanisms to maintain physical medicine control. One physiatrist stated that at some point "we are going to find some pretty powerful agitation for another medical professional organization—physical training, reconditioning, or call it what you will. And I do not think that this would be at all desirable or necessary from either an economic or professional standpoint."[133] In the VA economic competition was not an issue, and bureaucratic control made coordination possible. Yet, as we have seen, this control did not ensure coordination.

Disagreement among physiatrists over corrective therapy's role reflected different segments' views about the future course of their specialty (i.e., those who favored a broader conception of their work in reconditioning and rehabilitation versus those committed to the practice of physical medicine as their specialty's core task). Those who opposed extension of corrective therapy were predominant.

In the early 1950s, corrective therapists sought licensing legislation in Massachusetts and New York, as well as in several other states, to incorporate activities of daily living and ambulation training. Physical therapists quickly resisted and charged that "legal recognition [is] usually the last step in developing a profession [while] so far the first step—setting standards of education—had not been met by the corrective therapists."[134] They counterattacked by trying to convince physicians and legislators that the functions claimed by corrective therapy belonged to physical therapy. Physical therapy mobilized support for this campaign from its members and other groups,[135] and, as a result of these efforts and the lack of AMA and American Congress of Physical Medicine support, corrective therapy's licensing bills failed.

By obtaining licensing laws during the 1950s, physical therapy effectively blocked corrective therapists from establishing a foothold in civilian practice. For example, the uncertain legal situation of corrective therapy prevented Rusk from using the group in his Institute for Rehabilitation Medicine.[136] Only in New Mexico and Minnesota, where physical therapy laws are weak, has corrective therapy developed a significant civilian practice.[137]

In subsequent years corrective therapists unsuccessfully appealed to the American Congress of Physical Medicine[138] and to the AMA[139] for recognition and creation of accreditation mechanisms. The AMA, however, has not completely closed the door on corrective therapy; it has said that recognition might be granted if pathology courses were included in the corrective therapy curriculum. This has created dissension within corrective therapy about whether the group should stress its connections to medicine or physical education.[140] Lack of AMA acceptance has deprived corrective therapy of both a strong accreditation mechanism to structure its market and the legitimacy to gain recognition from such organizations as the NCA and the Office of Education. In addition, corrective therapists have failed to qualify for Medicare reimbursement.[141]

In the VA corrective therapy has experienced several threats to its survival. A merger with other occupational groups has even been suggested. Although they continue to occupy a shaky position, corrective therapists have maintained their independent occupational existence in the VA by developing an organization and a journal as well as political support from veterans groups.[142] They also have generally had the support of physiatrists in the VA, who have resisted efforts to consolidate the allied occupations within their domain. In 1970 there were 480 corrective therapists in the VA, compared to 497 physical therapists. However, there were 298 physical therapy assistants, while corrective therapy had only 39.[143]

In fact, attempts to deal with "overlapping functional responsibilities" in the Physical Medicine and Rehabilitation Service have been unsuccessful. In the 1966 administrative regulations detailing the functions of each occupational group, fifty-three functions were listed, twenty-two of which were shared by two or more occupations.[144] Reorganization of the central office in 1965 resulted in exclusion of all allied occupations. This met with a great deal of resistance from allied groups and veterans organizations.[145] In the early 1970s, representatives from the major allied groups were once again placed in the central office. In 1974 these representatives were from physical therapy, occupational therapy, and corrective therapy, with the possibility of others being added. These central office positions are important since the representative becomes an advocate for his or her group both inside and outside the VA. In short, efforts to consolidate occupations or to produce "generalist therapists" have not appreciably altered the existing division of labor. Once established, the occupations have resisted administrative challenges to their independent existence.

Physical Medicine and Rehabilitation at Midcentury

The early postwar years, particularly in the VA, mark the apex of physical medicine's power and prestige. Of course this does not mean they had a great deal of power or prestige relative to other specialties; in many ways they continued to struggle for recognition. Physical medicine entered the decade as a marginal segment and exited as a formally recognized specialty claiming expertise in "scientific management" of workers who provided rehabilitation services, not only through physical measures but through vocational, educational, and social ones as well. Rehabilitation work was incorporated as a core task within the context of war and its aftermath. During these years some physicians called for a separate residency program in rehabilitation, but this was unacceptable to the AMA Council on Physical Medicine and Council on Medical Education and Hospitals. Instead, the importance of this work to physical medicine was signified in 1949 by the addition of "rehabilitation" to the names of some institutions representing the specialty.[146]

Physical medicine and rehabilitation physicians also started emphasizing their expertise in the "scientific" diagnosis of problems, especially through electrical techniques such as electromyography.[147] These claims reflected the physiatrists' changing role and position in the medical division of labor. In this new role, the physiatrist did not usually provide treatment. The actual application of physical measures in therapy carried the aura of "dirty work." Instead, the physiatrist diagnosed the patient's ills and prescribed a therapeutic regimen administered by allied therapists under his control. This shift to claims based on scientific diagnosis and management was integrally associated with efforts by physical medicine physicians to place themselves strategically between other physicians and the allied occupations. Physiatrists claimed that their expertise in rehabilitation and their concept of treating the "whole man" made them sole authority when it came to the disabled and chronically ill, or the "third phase" of medicine.[148]

A by-product of this new strategic location in the hospital division of labor was that physiatrists became increasingly isolated from other members of their profession, whose acceptance they still sought. This isolation is seen by some as having exacerbated the problems of physical medicine and rehabilitation owing to a "lack of communication."[149] Because of this isolation and continued questioning of the physiatrist's expertise, physical medicine's position began to weaken in the 1950s.

For physical therapy and occupational therapy, the decade was one of rapid growth and solidification of their positions, under physician authority, in the medical division of labor. After the war physical therapists began a campaign for legal recognition from the states, reasoning that it was good to get a "law on the books while things are quiet."[150] In 1950 the APTA drafted a model law maintaining that the physical therapist would treat only "under the prescription, supervision, and direction of a person licensed to practice medicine and surgery."[151] This willingness to accept statutorily defined physician authority reflected concern about competition from corrective therapists and maverick physical therapists in New York.[152] The concern was not with physician dominance but with "trouble with cults, quacks, and 'commercials.'"[153] During the 1950s most states passed laws severely restricting these competitors.

One explanation for their licensing campaign is that it was partially motivated by a desire to gain autonomy from physicians. But the only indication of dissatisfaction was the suggestion by physical therapists that they should not confine themselves solely to the medical field; they should also investigate opportunities outside it. For example, one suggestion was to contact PTA presidents about opportunities in education.[154] That many people in the field now claim laws passed during this period more firmly tied the physical therapist to the physician suggests that autonomy from the medical profession was not their original intent.

While attaining such laws did help thwart competitors, their concern constituted a strategic error: competition from "cults and quacks" may not have been as significant a problem as it had been prior to the war. In establishing statutorily defined ties to the medical profession, they placed themselves in a difficult position in relation to what would become a very significant issue—attempts to establish some measure of autonomy.

During this period the APTA also linked a "firm public relations foundation" to the pursuit of licensing legislation.

The group developed contacts with fund-raising organizations such as the National Easter Seal Society and Community Chest, since they presented "ideal opportunities to tell the community about physical therapy."[155] The March of Dimes, for example, was asked to make sure that any photograph used in newspapers included a qualified physical therapist wearing an APTA emblem.[156] Also, the APTA's Interprofessional Relations Committee was mandated to establish connections and conduct a public relations campaign with other professional medical organizations.[157] They stressed the need for closer relations with other allied groups to provide "reciprocal assistance" in the legislative arena.[158] Through these activities, physical therapists created mechanisms to pursue their goals.

Although occupational therapists organized a Public Relations Committee and a Committee on Civil Service and Legislation to improve their "image" and statutory situation,[159] they did not match the zeal of physical therapists. They not only lacked resources to achieve legal recognition, they also sought to maintain the autonomy of their association. Although occupational therapists were unwilling to become subordinate to the medical profession, they did want to tie their services to the medical market. They argued strongly for the therapeutic nature of their work and tried to dissociate themselves from their earlier "arts and crafts" image. In fact, the AOTA recommended substituting the term "creative and manual skills" for the more usual "arts and crafts."[160]

Rather than become subordinate to medicine, occupational therapists sought to control their association by ending the tradition of filling the presidential post with a male from the medical profession. In 1947 the appointment of an occupational therapist as president of the AOTA broke this tradition. In the same year they published their own journal, *American Journal of Occupational Therapy* (AJOT), believing there was "little likelihood of the association obtaining professional stature without a truly representative publication."[161] The previous journal, *Occupational Therapy and Rehabilitation,* was continued under the editorship of Dr. Sidney Licht. Its focus, however, was on technical areas of interest to physiatrists and its title was eventually changed to *American Journal of Physical Medicine.*

To establish control over their professional activities, occupational therapists focused on internal matters. However, they did conduct publicity efforts through the National Society for Crippled Children and run fund-raising campaigns to improve their educational programs. Most important, they resisted attempts by physical medicine to extend control over their work and organization. For example, they described as "provocative" the suggestion that occupational therapy should be prescribed by a physiatrist,[162] and opposed efforts to appoint medical directors in occupational therapy schools. The occupational therapists favored the existing arrangement of medical direction through advisory committees, fearing control by a single medical specialty.[163]

The extent of their resistance to physical medicine's control should not be overemphasized. Occupational therapists questioned the degree of control physical medicine should have over their work, but were, along with the other allied occupations, more firmly under the authority of physical medicine and rehabilitation physicians than at any time in their history. Indeed, occupational therapy moved to ally itself more closely with the medical profession. The AMA's role in the training of occupational therapists as well as the importance of the physician's prescription were not questioned. "An ancillary, almost *handmaid of the Lord,* role seemed to be willingly accepted."[164]

By the middle of the twentieth century, physical medicine and rehabilitation physicians were at the top of an occupationally organized division of labor. Their authority derived from a complex of interlocking relationships formed during physical medicine's long struggle to gain a recognized share of the medical services market. While these relationships have since been severely tested, and consequently altered, they still influence the organization of rehabilitation work.

6

The Redivision of Labor, 1950–1980

Until the 1950s the allied occupations accepted their subordination to medicine because they perceived this relationship as beneficial and necessary. With the professionalization of groups such as chiropractors, and with the proliferation of new "therapy" workers such as corrective therapists, physical therapists wanted more protection of their territory than the medical profession provided. While physical therapists turned to state governments for protective licensing legislation, occupational therapists, for a variety of reasons, did not.

Since the mid-1950s the allied groups have tried to increase their autonomy vis-à-vis physical medicine and the medical profession. The enlarged federal role in health care during the 1960s created a more competitive market situation. Programs like Medicare and Medicaid and the Allied Health Act of 1966 supported the training of health workers and spurred the drive for autonomy by creating new service markets in hospitals, nursing homes, and home care.

By the early 1970s, however, various forces in the medical profession, the state, and the private sector aligned to prevent further increases in autonomy by allied occupations on the grounds that fragmentation had to be stopped. Nonetheless, physical therapists prevailed in this struggle and entered the 1980s with a secure and sizable market for their services. In fact they were so successful in the medical marketplace that other occupations have called the APTA to find how physical therapists accomplished this. By making a number of market mistakes since World War II, occupational therapists have been much less successful in their quest for autonomy.

The rise of allied occupations, especially physical therapy, in the rehabilitation division of labor has been paralleled by the fall of physical medicine as the dominant specialty in this area after World War II. Moves by physical therapists to assume increasing responsibility for treatment and diagnosis without dependence on physicians have not been countered by physiatrists. Attacks on physical medicine by other medical specialties have further weakened physiatrists' domain and control over rehabilitation work. For the most part, physiatrists assumed a defensive posture in the marketplace over the last thirty years and failed to develop a market approach that might have prevented their displacement in the division of labor, if not their possible demise in the future as a medical specialty.

Pursuit of Autonomy

The Rise of Physical Therapy

Beginning in 1946, the APTA encouraged legal recognition of the physical therapy profession through the enactment of physical therapy practice acts that would legally license or register therapists. The association furnished advice and guidance to the state chapters regarding legislative activity and encouraged its membership to take "an active and informed interest" in the state licensing issue.[1] "Sound ground work for future legislation" will only be laid, claimed the APTA president in 1951, if therapists "continue to give unsparingly of their time and energy. Protective legislation is vital if physical therapy is to progress!"[2]

Those state chapters which sought licensing faced opposition by traditional competitors, such as osteopaths, chiropractors, and masseurs, as well as by newer competitors, including naturopaths, reflexologists, herb dealers, and even some beauticians. To counter this opposition, and to increase the likelihood that state legislators would pass their bills, physical therapists sought the support of the more powerful lobby of state medical societies and nursing associations as well as private foundations such as the National Foundation for Infantile Paralysis and the Cerebral Palsy Association. In addition, physical therapists in some state chapters registered themselves as lobbyists, and in several states, lawyers, who were also legislators, were retained to sponsor physical therapy licensing legislation.[3]

In 1954 physical therapists demanded representation on medical examiners boards and an end to the requirement that certain medical specialties serve on the boards.[4] The former demand indicated a desire to gain influence vis-à-vis medicine, while the latter reflected a wish to alter physical medicine's control. The APTA called in 1957 for its local associations to press for state laws that would create "Boards of Physical Therapy Examiners" composed of two physical therapists and one physician. If this met with resistance, the APTA was willing to settle for an advisory group of physical therapists.[5]

By 1959, 31 states passed licensing laws for physical therapists.[6] Thirteen states had Boards of Physical Therapy (with 8 being composed entirely of physical therapists) and 18 had Boards of Medical Examiners (with 13 having advisory committees of physical therapists). A total of 15 states had "mandatory" laws that forbade use of the name "physical therapist" by anyone not meeting the association's requirements. The remaining 16 states had "permissive" laws that did not preclude the use of the name by other practitioners.[7] Only one state law made it possible to practice without physician prescription or supervision of physical therapy.

The AMA opposed the trend toward licensing and favored voluntary modes of registration. Licensing, according to them, should be pursued only when approved by organized medicine and jointly developed by the groups concerned.[8] Thus, the AMA created the Joint Committee to Study Para-Medical Areas in Relation to Medicine.[9] Later the name was changed to the Committee to Study the Relationships of Medicine with Allied Health Professions and Services, and it was given permanent status as the Department of Allied Medical Professions and Services. The committee was to study and make recommendations about the changing relationship of the allied groups to the medical profession. At its first meeting, the committee clearly demonstrated its support for the antilicensing policy of the AMA by commending the AOTA for establishing its own standards of practice through a registry.[10]

Physical therapists responded that the AMA was "rightfully afraid of allied fields starting independent practice," and noted that physical therapy was not among these fields. The APTA emphasized that the physical therapists were not moving away from the medical profession to compete with physicians in the fee-for-service market. They pointed to their increasingly complex relationships with organized medicine, and their belief that without the medical profession's support they would be left to the "mercy of chiropractors" and their "high-powered lobbyists."[11]

In the 1950s, APTA's Code of Ethics officially disapproved independent practice by physical therapists without "adequate and specific medical direction." Persons who practice "on their own," claimed one APTA president, "constitute a hazard to patient welfare since they are not prepared to diagnose nor are they qualified to determine what treatment a patient should receive."[12] Those therapists who disregarded this principle faced possible expulsion from the association. Of course expulsion from the APTA meant little unless state laws also prevented practice without referral from physicians, and not all states did this. In addition the association was careful to distinguish independent practitioners from "self-employed" physical therapists whose practices were "ethical" as long as they maintained "close relationships with referring physicians."[13]

Although the APTA to some extent lessened physical medicine's control in the 1950s, most licensing laws required a physician's prescription and thus prevented a move into the fee-for-service market. Rather than competing with physicians in the open market, physical therapists sought to make themselves "indispensable" to other medical specialties such as neurology and pediatrics at this time.[14] Thus, during the early 1960s, the APTA continued to support ties subordinating physical therapy to the medical profession. Despite the association's official policy, some physical therapists were starting to question the "direct supervision" of their work by physicians and to raise the possibility of private practice. As a result, two rival organizations were created: the National Association of Licensed Physical Therapists and the American Association of Independent Physical Therapists. Both promoted private practice in states without practice acts.

Physiatrists were concerned about this trend and pointed out that "some physical therapists do not understand the need for and resent medical supervision. Their training and their grasp of the practice of medicine has not been extensive enough for them to recognize their limitations."[15] Physiatrists were quick to emphasize that "self-employed" physical therapists, to whom patients were referred by a physician's prescription, must also have direct medical supervision as must physical therapists working in clinics.[16] In 1953 the American Congress of Physical Medicine and Rehabilitation and the American Society of Physical Medicine and Rehabilitation officially adopted the policy that "any therapist prescribing for and treating a patient on her knowledge rather than under the guidance of a physician presumes to have the medical judgment to practice medicine independently." Thus a physician's referral for treatment, according to physiatrists, no more covered a physical therapist assuming responsibility for treating a patient than it did a pharmacist dispensing a narcotic to a patient referred for a "pain killer."[17]

Such policy statements, however, had little effect on the growing movement within physical therapy for independent practice. Physiatrists were starting to fear that their position "as the inherent leader of the rehabilitation team" was being successfully challenged as some physical therapists "assumed leadership of the rehabilitation team." The *Archives* editorial continued:

> The physician has been erroneously placed in the position of consultant to the allied professions. . . . in their anxiety to establish personal stature, or to obtain professional recognition for reasons of sanctioning independent, private practices, they have lost sight of their proper roles as members of a coordinated team functioning in the best interests of a disabled patient.[18]

In his 1958 presidential address to the congress, Donald Rose spoke of the "tremendous upsurge of professionalistic spirit" in physical therapy, and commented: "I have grave doubts as to the ultimate value to us of this apparent course of events."[19] Rose concluded the address by calling on his colleagues to stop "giving away" the practice of medicine to allied occupations.[20] Other physiatrists believed that Rose's warning may have been too late. In their opinion, groups such as physical therapists were "eagerly panting for and in some instances actually succeeding in 'practising the healing arts,' etc."[21]

To reaffirm their control over physical therapists, physiatrists called for clarification of the extent and nature of their direction of physical therapy schools, as noted in the "Essentials." They maintained that medical directors should have direct contact on a day-to-day basis with physical therapists in training since they "are not likely to realize their relationship to the practice of medicine and the need for medical direction unless they actually experience medical direction throughout their training program." Physiatrists also opposed the practice in some schools of substituting for the director an advisory committee of representatives of various medical specialties who met a few times a year to give "medical direction" to the teaching program.[22]

These moves by physiatrists proved ineffective. Under pressure from the two new rival physical therapy organizations, and with federal subsidization of demand through Medicaid and Medicare, therapists started to enter the private practice market in the 1970s. While maintaining their official connection to the medical profession, physical therapists sought new state practice acts to permit greater autonomy.

For example, the New York law was successfully altered in 1974 to allow a physical therapist to practice with only a verbal diagnosis from a physician. The law originally required a written prescription, but this had been changed to an oral prescription in 1971. In California, no legally defined relationship existed between physical therapists and physicians, so therapists moved directly into the fee-for-service market to compete with physicians.[23]

Physicians were gravely concerned about the move by physical therapists to practice without a prescription. "This is in direct contravention of legal requirements which specify that only physicians may prescribe treatment for disease, pain, injury, or deformity," charged one physiatrist. He added that if physical therapists wanted to fight for permission to write prescriptions, "they must also then assume the responsibility for the effect of treatment which they have thus far been understandably reluctant to do, since this implies that any person could write an intelligent prescription based upon a diagnosis made by someone else."[24] Physical therapists angrily retorted that physicians had a "know-it-all attitude" toward the practice of medicine and refused to recognize the abilities of therapists.[25]

In 1982 the APTA officially adopted the policy that physical therapy practice would be independent of practitioner referral.[26] They even retained a law firm in Pittsburgh, Pennsylvania, to advise state chapters about changing licensing laws. By the early 1980s, six states passed new laws that allowed physical therapists to practice without a physician's referral. Although therapists were now allowed by law to practice independently in specific states, for all practical purposes they almost always needed a physician's referral to obtain third-party reimbursement. A major goal of physical therapists in the 1980s obviously will be to pressure third-party payers to drop requirements for physician referral.[27]

In addition to licensing, the APTA developed other mechanisms to improve its labor market. In 1955 it formed a joint committee with the AHA to revise the guidelines for accrediting hospital physical therapy departments and to examine the issue of medical direction of physical therapy.[28] Physical therapist resistance to the inclusion of occupational therapy on the joint committee reflects the importance they attached to this relationship with the AHA. The APTA wanted a separate committee to be established for occupational therapists, but the AHA refused.[29] The AOTA was denied this potentially favorable relationship for eight years, until such a committee was created in 1963.

Through this joint committee, physical therapists pressed hospitals to employ only fully qualified physical therapists and to restructure administrative and personnel policies.[30] While the AHA could enforce some of these policies and procedures, it was also necessary to get the Joint Committee on the Accreditation of Hospitals (JCAH) to accept and enforce any revised "Essentials," and the APTA therefore pressed them to rewrite the standards relating to physical therapy services in hospitals. Hopes for change were raised in 1968, when the JCAH took action to revise its standards. Two APTA members were asked to serve on a Physical Restorative Services Advisory Committee to discuss standards for a "physical restorative service" in a hospital. All other members of the thirteen-member committee were physicians, eight of whom were physiatrists.[31]

Discussion continued for eighteen months, with controversy centering on interpretations regarding medical direction of the physical therapy service, responsibility for administration, and the source of physical therapy prescriptions and referrals. The physical therapists also attacked the JCAH's references to their services as physical medicine services. Although the first draft of the committee's report referred to standards relative to physical therapy under the title "Physical Therapy Services," the final draft adopted by the JCAH carried physical therapy standards under the heading "Physical Medicine Services."

A "strongly worded letter" was sent to the JCAH from the APTA executive director protesting the mislabeling of physical therapy.[32] The APTA argued that physical medicine represented a recognized medical specialty, and it did not want to be identified only with physiatrists or seen as a "subsidiary component" of physical medicine. Rather, the APTA maintained that physical therapy was a service used by a variety of specialties. They also pointed out that the JCAH's substitution of "Physical Medicine Services" for "Physical Therapy Services" in the 1971 hospital accreditation manual completely disregarded the fact that most hospitals did not have physical medicine departments.[33]

In short, the JCAH's action was seen by the APTA as an overt attempt to "interpose the physiatrist between the physical therapist and other referring practitioners." Thus the JCAH was supporting "a philosophy of autonomous medical control" by physical medicine over all rehabilitative services in hospitals.[34] One APTA president claimed that the JCAH "has been attempting to force domination and control of physical therapy services by physical medicine and rehabilitation."[35] Further evidence, according to the APTA, of the committee's attempt to reinforce the control of physiatrists over physical therapists in hospitals could be seen in the composition of the Physical Medicine Services Advisory Committee, created in 1972 by the JCAH to consider further revisions of the standards. Twenty-nine physiatrists, eight other physicians, primarily orthopedists, three physical therapists, and one occupational therapist comprised this advisory committee. In addition to being vastly outnumbered, the representatives from the APTA and AOTA did not serve as official committee members.[36] In 1977 the APTA was still unable to influence JCAH physical therapy standards.

Physical therapists also tried to end use of the registry developed in 1935 by the American Congress of Physical Medicine to control entry into physical therapy. Physiatrists opposed this move, claiming that the registry was "appreciated and encouraged by farsighted and ethical therapists, since it was a factor which helped elevate them to a professional level."[37] This led to the formation in 1958 of an ad hoc committee representing the APTA, the American Congress of Physical Medicine and Rehabilitation, and the American Registry for Physical Therapy. After the ad hoc committee failed to maintain registry use, a permanent liaison committee was established between the APTA, AHA, the Congress, and the American Academy of Physical Medicine and Rehabilitation (formerly the American Society of Physical Medicine and Rehabilitation).[38] In 1965 the congress also sought assistance from the AMA Council on Medical Education and Hospitals to reestablish use of the registry for physical therapists, but the council refused to intervene.[39] In fact, previous efforts by the council to bring the conflicting parties together had been unsuccessful.[40] Having obtained licensing legislation in most states, the physical therapists no longer needed physical medicine's registry.

A further effort by physical therapists was directed toward wresting control over accreditation from the AMA's Council on Medical Education and Hospitals. In 1955 a compromise revision of the "Essentials of an Acceptable School of Physical Therapy" was reached by the APTA and the AMA Council on Medical Education and Council on Physical Medicine and Rehabilitation. By 1960 a "collaborative" process of accreditation was begun which provided for APTA representation on the accrediting bodies.[41] However, the Council on Medical Education did not recognize the APTA as coequal with the AMA in the collaborative accreditation process; the AMA was recognized as the accrediting body and the APTA as the collaborative organization. Thus, while the APTA gained representation on the accrediting bodies, the AMA for the most part still had unilateral decision-making power over educational programs in physical therapy, as established in the revised 1955 "Essentials."

In 1967 the APTA unsuccessfully applied to the NCA for independent accrediting status. (NCA, the nongovernmental body of accrediting agencies, is the predecessor of the Commission on Postsecondary Accreditation, or COPA.) In 1971 the NCA declared a moratorium on recognizing new agencies to prevent further fragmentation of accrediting bodies pending completion of the Study of Accreditation of Selected Health Education Programs (SASHEP). The SASHEP commission report, released in 1972, recommended creation of a national council on accreditation. While allied health professions strongly supported this proposal, physicians rejected it because AMA accreditation practices would have come under scrutiny as well.[42] The APTA also failed to gain recognition from the federal accrediting body, the U.S. Office of Education (USOE).[43] In 1974 the APTA again unsuccessfully pursued independent accrediting status for physical therapist and physical therapy assistant educational programs, as part of its newly revised "Essentials." The AMA rejected this idea because the revision did not require physician direction of physical therapy educational programs and failed to mention limitations on the practice of physical therapy. In addition, approval was denied because some physical therapy curricula included instruction in electromyography. One AMA official rejected this version of the APTA's revised "Essentials" because if adopted, they would, in his opinion, condone the independent practice of medicine by physical therapists without physician control. Another AMA representative objected on the grounds that they would probably create the "chiropractors of the future."[44]

Charles Magistro, in his 1975 APTA presidential address, responded to these charges. Educational programs in physical therapy, he claimed, had to be directed by physical therapists because they, rather than physicians, were the experts in this field. The charge that the latest "Essentials" did not indicate limitations in physical therapy practice simply had no basis, according to Magistro, because individual state licensing laws regulated such practice. As for the AMA's concern over electromyography instruction in physical therapy curricula, Magistro pointed out that this technique was not even mentioned in the "Essentials" and that responsibility for performance of this procedure rested with individual state boards of medical examiners.[45]

Revisions proposed by the AMA in 1975 were unacceptable to the APTA because it felt that continued attempts were being made to regulate the practice of physical therapy through its educational standards. At the same time, USOE and COPA again reaffirmed the right of the AMA Council on Medical Education and Hospitals to accredit physical therapy educational programs. Frustrated by repeated failures to assume their own accrediting powers, APTA members began to call for severing their "feudal-plebian relationship" with the AMA, at least with regard to accreditation.[46] The 1976 APTA presidential address even raised the possibility that the association would simply terminate, unilaterally, its collaborative arrangement with the AMA.[47]

In early 1977 the APTA again requested independent accrediting status from USOE and COPA. Their decision was to recognize temporarily two accrediting bodies, one from the APTA and one from the AMA. The APTA saw this as a partial success; now its goal was to become the only accrediting agency for physical therapy. Therapists, however, feared "continued coercion" by the AMA to limit the APTA's accrediting activities.[48] Backed by the AHA and the American Society of Allied Health Professions (ASAHP), the AMA opposed recognition of the APTA and tried to discredit its newly acquired accrediting status.[49] The AMA not only failed to do this, it lost USOE recognition in 1979 as an accrediting agency for physical therapy training programs. The AMA continued to be recognized by the voluntary body, COPA, and therefore remained involved in accreditation, but no longer in collaboration with the APTA.

The allied occupations now felt "tuned to the efforts to manipulate our acquiescence with both imperceptible subtlety and overt obstructionism."[50] Thus, the APTA was "concerned" about a proposed Conference to Consider Issues in the Accreditation of Allied Health Education, cosponsored by ASAHP, COPA, USOE, and the Bureau of Health Manpower in 1979. Noting that the steering committee for the conference had only two members from the allied health field, and none from physical therapy, the APTA president wrote to the steering committee requesting a broadening of representation.[51] At least when it came to accreditation of educational programs, physical therapists would no longer tolerate the "father-knows-best" approach of medicine. The final tie was broken in 1983 with the AMA withdrawal from COPA. Physicians continue to serve on accreditation site visit teams, but at the behest of APTA.[52]

To many within the allied health field, APTA's termination of its collaboration with the AMA signified a break in the AMA's long history of dominance over allied health occupations. Physical therapists had now laid a foundation that would allow them to depose physiatrists as the controlling occupation in the rehabilitation division of labor.

Occupational Therapy's Market Mistakes

In contrast to physical therapists, occupational therapists did not pursue licensing legislation until the 1970s. They instead developed strong internal certification mechanisms at the national level to control entry while avoiding further subordination to medicine. Indeed, in the 1950s, the AOTA feared that some physical therapy licensing bills might force occupational therapy into the control of physiatrists. In Connecticut, for example, occupational therapists were worried about the inclusion of occupational therapy in a bill presented before the state legislature to license physical therapists. The opening paragraph of the Connecticut bill mentioned occupational therapy: "Physical Medicine is composed of physical therapy and occupational therapy." Occupational therapists claimed that even this brief mention of their field would have led to their licensing, and that it was introduced to the state legislature before the local AOTA chapter knew anything about it.[53] To support its state chapter's opposition to this bill, the national office of the AOTA officially opposed licensure that year. The bill was soon withdrawn.

Occupational therapists continued to oppose licensure through the 1960s. They believed that licensure "made you a second-class citizen," and that voluntary certification "was the classy way to go" because it entailed self-governance[54] and prevented further subordination to the medical profession.[55] Licensure was something you would obtain, they argued, if you were an electrician, plumber, or beautician, but not if you were a member of a developing profession. Thus, the AOTA was adamant that the APTA was wrong to pursue licensing legislation. In addition, occupational therapists believed that state licensure would be a deterrent to moving one's practice to other states, would not guarantee protection of patients, and would require continuing safeguards to prevent pressure groups from effecting amendments that might lower the standards of the AOTA.[56]

Failure to organize a local political base to pursue licensing legislation meant that occupational therapists could not take advantage of opportunities arising in the late 1960s. For example, they were unable to influence Medicare legislation, although physical and speech therapists, with licensing and a stronger political base, could do so.[57] As a result, Medicare reimbursed occupational therapists for hospital care only if physical therapy, speech therapy, or nursing was the primary service. Thus, occupational therapy became dependent on other allied occupations for reimbursement, since it could not by law be the sole provider of service.[58]

The AOTA's failure to have a representative in Washington, D.C., until 1968 demonstrated its lack of readiness for the expanded federal role.[59] Since then, the AOTA has moved its headquarters to Washington, and replaced many of the occupational therapists on its staff with experts in public relations and lobbying. Those remaining are concerned with internal matters such as education and certification.[60] AOTA's most significant action was to form a Government Affairs Department to watch legislative events and to develop strategies for utilizing political channels. A couple of years after the founding of the American Physical Therapy Congressional Action Committee (APTCAC), the AOTA authorized the formation of a political action committee in 1976, and started funding it in 1978.[61] Like APTCAC, the American Occupational Therapy Political Action Committee (AOTPAC) solicited voluntary contributions from members to be directly channeled into the election campaigns of political candidates who might support or push health care legislation favorable to occupational therapy. In its first year, AOTPAC supported 29 candidates for federal office in 22 states, thus putting "[its] foot firmly in the door."[62]

Another reason for the AOTA's unreadiness for the expanded role of the federal government is that its commodity was either unknown or misunderstood by politicians, health professionals, and the general public. Frequent *AJOT* editorials in the early 1960s pointed out the frustration and embarrassment of occupational therapists "stumbling back and forth" to define their work.[63] "'Just what does an occupational therapist do?' Most of us hear this question or variations of it all too frequently. Do you sigh helplessly, 'It's too complicated to explain right now,' launch into a carefully prepared dissertation or say vaguely 'Oh you know . . .' and let the conversation drift to other subjects?"[64] Another editorial commented: "The usual reaction to any mention of the 'OT Image' is either a low moan or a pained 'oh no, not again.'"[65] Even the AOTA's Committee on Clinical Practice, whose primary function in 1963 was to define occupational therapy, was unsuccessful in this task.[66]

The 1965 AOTA presidential address expressed concern over this problem of definition because it was thought to cause underutilization of the field by physicians.[67] Over a decade later another AOTA president again made the same observation. She noted at least one physician who said: "You know, doctors are stupid: they don't understand occupational therapy. If you walked down the hall of a hospital and asked 50 doctors what occupational therapy is, you might find one that could tell you but I doubt it."[68]

To improve the demand for services and "achieve success in marketing them," occupational therapists started calling for clearer and more positive identification of their product.[69] Occupational therapists now sought "to transform" the meaning of their work into "an identifiable, describable, recognizable, and valued commodity."[70] AOTA leaders compared this task to that of developing and marketing any new product, and told their membership that an approach like that used in the business world had to be adopted "to build a consistent public image."[71]

Thus public relations efforts were to focus not just on the lay public but on physicians and third-party payers such as Blue Cross, and insurance companies such as Home and Prudential.[72] In 1975, for example, occupational therapists were insulted by a comment made in a *Time* film review. Film critic Jay Cocks stated in the last line of his review of *Front Page*: "this is a movie conceived with indifference and made with disinterest like a piece of occupational therapy."[73] AOTA's legal counsel, in a letter to *Time*, called this remark a "flippant put-down."[74] A five-year "master plan" was even proposed in 1979 to educate the public and professionals through the use of TV, radio, national magazine ads, billboards, fliers and brochures.[75]

To improve the definition of their commodity, occupational therapists redefined the nature of their work to deemphasize a connection to medicine. Although this connection has not been completely severed, and probably will not be, some leaders in the field have criticized their dependence on the medical model and the medical profession. For example, one prominent occupational therapist writes that her field has "uncritically accepted close ties with medicine."[76] Adoption of the disease approach, she notes, "is ill-suited to our practice and . . . has interfered with our thinking. Perhaps education would provide a more useful model."[77] Similarly, the president of AOTA in 1973 claimed that when occupational therapy tries to influence the "pathological process," it "loses sight of man as a whole" and makes occupational therapists doubt "the viability of occupational therapy."[78]

Occupational therapists have not sought to dissociate completely from medicine per se but to break the control physicians have over them by redefining their work.[79] One way in which they did this was to question the traditional definition of their work as "medically prescribed." In the early 1960s, therapists in the area of psychiatric occupational therapy challenged the requirement of a physician's prescription. Calling it "anachronistic," occupational therapists argued that the prescription hindered communication, oversimplified the therapist's experience, and confined the occupational therapist's role to that of a "technical assistant."[80]

Soon occupational therapists also questioned the use of the prescription in areas outside of psychiatry. While the prescription was often followed superficially in actual practice,[81] the real objection to the prescription was that it limited the "professional growth" of occupational therapy.[82] In 1962 the words "medically prescribed" were deleted from the definition of occupational therapy as it appeared in the AOTA Fact Sheet.[83] Commenting on this deletion, one therapist remarked that the AOTA no longer wanted to define itself as the use of "medically prescribed activities." She noted that the prescription was a "concrete symbol" of occupational therapy's "authoritative-dependent relationship" with physicians, and as such, it had to end.[84] For years physicians had objected to proposals to end the written prescription of occupational therapy. In the words of one physiatrist, the written prescription was "basic and very necessary," and any therapist who did not follow it carefully exercised "poor judgment."[85]

Another way in which occupational therapists deemphasized their connection to medicine was by developing a new theoretical base drawn from the behavioral sciences. Occupational therapists could have a foundation rooted in medicine, claimed one AOTA president, and still not be "subservient to physicians" or forced to work only in hospitals.[86] Thus, their goal in the late 1970s was to develop a theoretical base entailing some "necessary relationship to medicine without restricting [them] to dependency within that relationship."[87] By partially disengaging from medicine and rehabilitation, occupational therapists have tried to define a unique role for themselves. They have returned to their nineteenth-century roots in "moral treatment."[88] One physician proponent of occupational therapy recently stated that "a new era of moral treatment tailored to our times is sorely needed."[89] Using modern scientific terms, they have portrayed this as an evolution of a higher-order theoretical base founded in neurology, biology, and psychology.[90] Even suggestions for a new name, such as occupational behaviorists, occupational scientists, developmental scientists, and life skill specialists, have been made to dissociate from the medical model.[91]

Occupational therapists have thus come full circle in defining their work. Clearly, changes in this definition have not resulted from natural evolution of the field, but from the competitive market situation faced by occupational therapy. These attempts to improve commodity definition, however, have only further muddled the nature of occupational therapy services. Little consensus exists today, even within the occupation, as to what really distinguishes its expertise from other groups.

Moreover, efforts by occupational therapists to clarify and improve the definition of their services have not focused their expertise; it has been diffused over a variety of new work settings. Some occupational therapists fear their colleagues might be overextending themselves, perhaps due "to the inherent gypsy in us."[92] Such overextension, suggested one AOTA special committee, might destroy any "commonalty of purpose, theories, and values" in occupational therapy, making it an umbrella term for a collection of specialty groups.[93] Others pointed out that such expansion constituted an invasion of a number of groups, "starting with a nursery school teacher up to and including a marriage counselor, as well as some of the things which a lawyer might do from time to time."[94]

Occupational therapy's new theoretical foundation provided a rationale for broadening the responsibilities of occupational therapists. In the early 1970s, they started to move beyond their traditional market in hospitals. New settings considered or actually moved into included nursing homes, schools, patients' homes and workplaces, prisons, community health agencies, and day care centers.[95] By criticizing the narrowness of the acute-care model of medicine, occupational therapists also used their new theoretical base as a justification for providing health education, preventive care, care for the terminally ill, and "socioenvironmental interventions in the general community."[96]

This expansiveness forced occupational therapists to distinguish themselves from competing groups in social work, psychology, and nursing, and from newer groups stressing the use of art, dance, and music. It was important for occupational therapists to distinguish their expertise from that of competitors to ensure continued employment in settings where they faced increased competition by workers who seemed to practice some variant of occupational therapy, sometimes at less cost to the employer. Yet occupational therapists have not been very successful at this. For example, as early as 1962 occupational therapists were concerned about the overlap of their own work with that of activity and recreational therapists, and made several attempts to clarify the differences.

Especially in psychiatric and geriatric settings, activity and recreational therapists claimed to provide "diversional" and "leisure time activities" that greatly overlapped with services provided by occupational therapists.[97] A "poor activity program," noted an occupational therapist, was activity therapy, while "a good one" was occupational therapy. Elaborating this distinction, she maintained that activity therapy was "designed for participation, but not specifically for ego involvement." Since, in her opinion, activity therapy appealed to the "automatic, learned patterns of behavior," it tended to "deny the dignity of a human being to struggle, to control his environment," "make man quiescent within the hospital community" and "depersonalize, institutionalize and, in general, debase human nature." Occupational therapy, however, "makes the assumption that the mind and will of man are occupied through central nervous system action and that man can and should be involved consciously in problem solving and creative activity."[98]

Occupational therapists continued to distinguish their competencies from those of activity and recreational therapists. In the late 1960s, occupational therapists objected to the language of Medicare amendments, which put diversionary and recreational activities under the direction of an occupational therapist. The AOTA legislation committee recommended that this language be changed to indicate that "appropriate diversionary and recreational activities may be given consultation by a qualified occupational therapist," as well as by a social worker or nurse. The committee explained that direction of diversional programs was not the role of an occupational therapist because occupational therapy was a medical, not a recreational, service.[99]

The AOTA reconsidered the state licensing issue in the early 1970s to gain a more favorable market position and enhance their political influence. Several AOTA chapters started agitating for licensing that would limit use of the title "occupational therapist." They wanted to take advantage of new third-party reimbursement possibilities in addition to Medicare;[100] only by restricting the performance of certain tasks to occupational therapists and by requiring institutions receiving federal funds to provide occupational therapy services could they do this.

In 1968, Puerto Rico was the first AOTA chapter to obtain a licensing law for registered occupational therapists and certified occupational therapy assistants. In the opinion of one observer, occupational therapists in Puerto Rico viewed licensure "as a means of obtaining priority for employment, security, and equal status with the physical therapists at a time when great emphasis and a large expenditure of funds were being granted for work with the older population."[101] As early as 1972 occupational therapists in New York and Florida started considering the licensure issue.[102] The New York chapter was particularly concerned about a recent Alabama court decision that established minimum constitutional standards for the mentally ill, but did not include occupational therapists as qualified mental health professionals because they were unlicensed. Moreover, this decision was cited as a national precedent and affected occupational therapists in New York as well as Pennsylvania, Kansas, and elsewhere.[103]

State associations such as New York's played a vital role in changing AOTA's attitude toward licensure. In 1974 the position of AOTA on licensure was officially changed from neutrality to endorsement, and "the pursuit of licensure was advanced to an objective with high priority."[104] In the following year, both New York and Florida enacted occupational therapy licensure bills.

Yet by 1982 only twelve more states and the District of Columbia were able to enact occupational therapy practice acts. Opposition primarily came from unlicensed competitors, such as recreation and activity therapists, and to a lesser degree, from art and music therapists.[105] Unlicensed competitors opposed the occupational therapists because of the fear they would "lose certain prerogatives." Some opposition from licensed competitors, such as physical therapists, arose because of "potential limitations" for them in occupational therapy practice acts.[106] Moreover, many states developed an "adverse legislative attitude" toward licensure because of growing support for the HEW licensure moratorium.[107] Further compounding the problem for occupational therapists were commissions created by many states to review new licensure proposals outside the usual political arena. Members of these commissions usually were not elected officials, and therefore could not be politically pressured in the same manner as legislators.[108]

These overall efforts by AOTA to increase their political influence and improve their commodity definition were largely aimed at changing Medicare regulations, especially those that made occupational therapy dependent on other allied occupations for reimbursement. They sought support from the AMA, the AHA, and the National Easter Seal Society for occupational therapy as an independent service in Medicare law, rather than as "an arm or sub-system of physical therapy." The association exhorted its members to take "aggressive action" to change Medicare law language that "hid" occupational therapy under physical therapy in Medicare programs, "thus distorting public identity of occupational therapy as a separate service and skewing utilization figures upward for physical therapy and downward for occupational therapy."[109] Occupational therapists were frustrated by this reimbursement policy, which they saw as discriminatory. "This situation can no longer be tolerated," remarked one therapist. It was unfair, she noted, that by law an occupational therapist even with a master's degree was not considered competent to be a primary health provider.[110]

In addition to trying to get themselves written into Medicare law as primary providers, occupational therapists sought to extend the coverage of their services to include outpatient care. AOTA president Jerry Johnson went so far as to proclaim that "unless occupational therapists solve the gigantic problems of reimbursement for our services, we shall cease to exist." As examples, she cited two occupational therapy departments, one that was not referred patients by its own medical staff because there was "no way to recoup the cost of service" and another that was firing its occupational therapy staff because it could not pay their salaries. In 1976 Johnson called on her association to begin "extremely urgent, skillful, consistent negotiations" with politicians, the federal government, and the AMA to "preserve our profession." She warned that it may "already be too late, and there will be resistance from other professions who themselves being already secure in the knowledge of their own reimbursement eligibility will be anything but eager to share the limited amounts of money available to pay for health care."[111]

Despite Johnson's plea for a grass roots campaign and the use of lobbyists to pressure politicians,[112] the AOTA repeatedly failed to have an amendment passed that would expand Medicare coverage for outpatient occupational therapy services and remove the need for nursing, physical therapy, or speech therapy as a condition for coverage. Occupational therapists have achieved a change in the original requirement that one of the "primary" services be ongoing for occupational therapy to be reimbursed. Now the primary service can be terminated and occupational therapy can continue as the sole service.

The failure to eliminate their dependent situation in Medicare legislation made occupational therapists especially wary of national health insurance proposals made during the Nixon Administration which would authorize the same coverage for occupational therapy as the Medicare program.[113] AOTA quickly responded to the three national health insurance bills in Congress by calling them "inadequate" and insisting that any national health insurance legislation include occupational therapy as a primary service both in hospital and outpatient settings.[114] The association soon gained support for the inclusion of occupational therapy services in national health insurance legislation from organizations such as the National Easter Seal Society, the American Congress of Rehabilitation Medicine, and the International Association of Rehabilitation Facilities.[115]

In the late 1970s, AOTA also sought to improve its third-party reimbursement by convincing private insurance companies and large insurance purchasers that occupational therapy was a necessary, appropriate, and cost-effective health care service. In 1977 the Health Insurance Association of America recommended to its 350 member companies inclusion of occupational therapy services in health benefit plans when referred by a physician.[116] Following up on this recommendation, in 1978 AOTA contacted eleven of the largest insurance companies to encourage coverage of occupational therapy services.[117]

These moves by occupational therapists to improve their market position have been far less successful than those of physical therapists. Their earlier failure to pursue licensing legislation and to define their commodity meant that they could not take advantage of the enlarged federal role in the 1960s and early 1970s. Recent attempts to remedy previous market mistakes have been, at best, only modestly successful. Their commodity still is uncertain; occupational therapists in the 1980s continue to agonize over the "reigning ambiguity" of their field. Late pursuers of licensing laws, occupational therapists encountered substantial resistance that they were not politically organized to defeat. Occupational therapists remain unlicensed in many states; even when licensed, they are not able to practice independently. Unless occupational therapists can correct their course in the rehabilitation marketplace, they will remain subordinated to other groups in the division of labor.

The Fall from Power

Marginality and Supply Problems

Physiatry reached its peak in the early 1950s. The Baruch Committee announced its dissolution in 1951 because its goals had been achieved: physiatry was recognized as a specialty through the creation of a Physical Medicine and Rehabilitation Section in the AMA and an American Board of Physical Medicine and Rehabilitation to control entry into the specialty. An academic presence for physiatry was crafted by funding residency fellowships, as well as major training and research centers at universities. Demand outside academic centers was promoted by the establishment of community rehabilitation centers. And even a scientific base was molded by supporting research and publication by physiatrists.[118]

Physiatrists like Krusen spoke encouragingly about the specialty's progress. "It is obvious," he wrote, "that the scope of our new medical discipline is enormous and that the future of our specialty is promising. Our recent progress has been truly phenomenal and this field . . . should attain new heights in this 'age of physics.'"[119] Other physiatrists called this postwar period a "renaissance in Physical Medicine."[120]

Although physiatrists created a demand for rehabilitation, they were unable to change the marginal image of their specialty. "The medical profession as a whole still shows discouragingly little interest in this field," claimed a 1952 *Archives* editorial.[121] Even during physical medicine's peak, physiatrists of Rusk's stature had trouble drawing an audience when the topic of discussion was rehabilitation. Rusk recalls that he was lucky if a dozen physicians attended his talks when the word "rehabilitation" was in the title. "These, more often than not, were the 'captive' audience invited by the host to dinner preceding the meeting and a number who attended because they had no other place to go." To attract more people, he retitled his talks "Dynamic Therapeutics in Chronic Disease." A number of physicians would then come "because they thought I had discovered a new type of vitamin or injection and they wanted to get in on the ground floor."[122] The persistent lack of "professional enthusiasm" shown by the medical profession toward physical medicine and rehabilitation[123] was manifested in the booklet *Functions and Structure of a Modern Medical School.*[124] Published by the AMA's Council on Medical Education and Hospitals in 1957, this booklet failed to disclose any reference to the term "physical medicine and rehabilitation" or its place in medical education. Similarly, physiatry was not represented on President Kennedy's 1962 Panel on Mental Retardation, even though many mentally retarded patients seen in rehabilitation settings had neuromuscular problems treated by physiatrists.[125]

Marginality continued to be a problem. In 1978 the White House Conference on Employment of the Handicapped underscored physiatry's image as a "diagnostically unchallenging field, requiring long-term therapy commitments and yielding little success."[126] A recent *JAMA* editorial failed to include physical medicine and rehabilitation among twenty-five specialties and subspecialties.[127] One physiatrist, assessing the "viability" of his specialty in the 1980s, sadly remarked:

> To be blunt, it is much easier to obtain visibility and acceptance with academic colleagues and medical students as a specialist in sports medicine or in the diagnosis and management of ambulatory patients with muscle diseases, than as a manager of rehabilitation services to the same patients.[128]

Physiatry's marginality resulted in a perpetual undersupply of workers. The existence of only 300 certified physiatrists by 1955 "strongly suggests not only a lagging interest in this field but the urgent necessity for active recruitment."[129] Attempts to recruit more physicians into physiatry have consistently failed. In 1949, for example, 0.35 percent of physicians entering residency training chose physical medicine and rehabilitation. In the mid-1950s, only 48 percent of the residency programs in physical medicine and rehabilitation were filled (compared to 80 percent in all residencies), and courses in physical medicine were typically enrolled far below those of other specialties.[130] According to an AMA survey, physical medicine got the lowest rating of all fields of practice in total course hours offered and physician hours of attendance between 1952 and 1955. During this period only 0.6 percent of all physicians surveyed expressed interest in instruction in physical medicine and rehabilitation.[131] By 1957 the specialty attracted 0.5 percent of graduating physicians, and was still the least popular medical specialty next to proctology, which attracted 0.43 percent of the first-year residents.[132]

In the 1960s and 1970s the academic presence of physical medicine and rehabilitation declined even further from its tenuous position of the 1950s. Not only did many four-year medical schools lack approved residency programs in physical medicine, over one-quarter of the medical schools did not even have a program in this specialty in the mid-1960s.[133] The number of approved residencies dropped from a high of 115 in 1963 to 69 a decade later, and stayed at about this level through the 1970s.[134] In the same period, the proportion of foreign medical graduates (FMGs) in university-affiliated residency programs, an inverse indicator of the status and popularity of a specialty, increased from 29 to 62 percent. When all residency programs in physical medicine and rehabilitation are examined for this period, the proportion of FMGs increased by 360 percent.[135]

In the 1970s, physiatry remained an unpopular specialty choice. In 1976, of the 21,145 physicians in the first year of residency training, only 166 were trained in physical medicine.[136] This number dropped even further by 1980, to 90.[137] The effect of such poor recruitment during the postwar years meant that few physicians practicing in university or non-university settings were certified physiatrists. Specifically, only 0.5 percent of all physicians (900 out of 180,000) in specialty practice in 1980 were in physical medicine and rehabilitation.[138] Thus, in terms of manpower requirements, physiatry has not kept supply in line with the demand it helped to create.

Market Challenges

To overcome their marginality, physiatrists tried to convince other physicians that their methods were clinically effective and that their practice was intellectually and financially rewarding. However, this posture has not allowed physiatrists to obtain closure around a specific body of knowledge and an assortment of techniques. Without such closure physiatrists have found it difficult to persuade physicians that physical medicine and rehabilitation has methods and a mission worthy of specialty status. In addition, this strategy only served to open physiatry's domain to other specialties on its boundary.

The biggest incursion into physiatrists' claimed expertise has been by orthopedic surgeons. In the mid-1950s, the latter staked a claim to "rehabilitation" and forestalled physical medicine's desire to control other physicians' use of physical and occupational therapists. The orthopedic surgeons submitted resolutions to the AMA's House of Delegates in 1953 to restrict use of the term "rehabilitation," and to prevent physiatrists from serving as advisors to the Council on Medical Education and Hospitals, which developed standards for physical and occupational therapy.[139] The orthopedic surgeons held that they were responsible for the development of these allied occupations and should therefore be involved in setting standards of education and rules of activity. After two years of meetings by a special committee appointed to study the matter, the Council on Physical Medicine and Rehabilitation became the "Council on Rehabilitation," with participation by all interested specialties. The word "Rehabilitation" was dropped from the Section on Physical Medicine and Rehabilitation (the stated purpose being that the Section on Physical Medicine and the Section on Orthopedic Surgery would develop joint sessions on rehabilitation). To replace the transformed council, a new Council on Medical Physics was created which would be concerned only with standardizing and certifying medical equipment.[140]

Physiatrists like academy president William Benham Snow described this "jurisdictional dispute" as "a matter of semantics."[141] If physiatrists were to be faulted at all for this "unhappy incident," Snow claimed, it would only be for their "enthusiasm, singleness of purpose, and vigor." He predicted in 1954 that this "challenge" from "our nearest relation" would soon pass.[142]

The dispute with orthopedic surgery proved to be more serious and long-lived than Snow estimated. Within a couple of years physiatrists were referring to their dispute with orthopedic surgery as a "battle."[143] They claimed that orthopedists were taking over their professional role. "Many orthopedists," remarked a leader in the physical medicine field, "consider themselves better qualified to prescribe exercise for their patients than are the physiatrists at their hospitals."[144]

Orthopedic surgeons were beginning to move into the rehabilitation area. Disturbed by what they perceived as a loss of patients to physiatrists in the 1950s, orthopedists called for the development within their specialty of rehabilitation programs that would include physical medicine.[145] Orthopedists actively promoted the idea of "orthopedic medicine" or "non-surgical orthopedics," which would be indistinguishable from physical medicine and rehabilitation. Patterned after phys-iatrists, nonsurgical orthopedists would treat patients by the physical agents of heat, light, massage, hydrotherapy, and electricity; teach special exercises and activities of daily living; and "do whatever is necessary for the restoration of the pa-tient to maximum function and usefulness at home and in employment, using all forms of therapy now used by the specialist in physical medicine and rehabilitation."[146]

In 1962 the president of the American Academy of Or-thopedic Surgeons thanked physiatrists for "stirring up" or-thopedists' interest in rehabilitation and referred to "orthopedic rehabilitation" as an "attractive opportunity for orthopedists with proper motivation and ability to feature nonoperative orthopedics as a subspecialty." Such orthopedic subspecialists would "care for non-surgical and orthopedic patients and par-ticipate in postoperative management when complex, pro-tracted rehabilitation techniques are needed." A specialist trained in orthopedic rehabilitation, it was argued, "would be eminently prepared to preside over a rehabilitation center" as "captain" of the team.[147] The call by orthopedists for the creation of a subspecialty of orthopedic rehabilitation culmi-nated in 1968 when the American Orthopedic Association formed a Rehabilitation Section.

The greater concern of physiatrists was that orthopedists might gain control over physical and occupational therapists, "for if that should happen, the physical medicine specialist would become less than a foreman; he would become a clerk."[148] Orthopedic surgeons pointed to the "strained rela-tionship" between physiatry and physical and occupational therapy, and the fact that many therapy schools objected to direction by physiatrists. Orthopedists opposed physiatrists directing schools for therapists on the grounds that these allied specialties were originally developed by orthopedic sur-geons, and that these therapies involved treatment by phys-ical means which orthopedists also used.[149] In the 1950s orthopedic surgeons succeeded in becoming administratively

responsible for physical and occupational therapy departments in some hospitals.

Also, in the late 1950s and early 1960s, orthopedic surgeons
established themselves in some medical schools as chairs of
physical medicine and rehabilitation training programs.[150] Indeed some of these programs only had orthopedists on the
faculty, leading physiatrists to call for their appointment to
medical school faculties "to ensure that the programs for training in physical medicine and rehabilitation . . . will not be
curtailed by other specialties."[151] Other medical schools, such
as the one at the University of California, San Francisco, organizationally placed physical medicine and rehabilitation as
a section under orthopedic surgery, with physiatrists directly
accountable to orthopedists.[152]

Orthopedists began to question whether physical medicine
and rehabilitation was a legitimate medical specialty. They
claimed that orthopedic surgeons used physical methods in
the treatment of patients having musculoskeletal disease years
before physical medicine and rehabilitation became a specialty. Physiatry only came about, orthopedists maintained,
as a "marriage of convenience" after World War II. "The physicians limiting their work to rehabilitation were few and, in
reality, rehabilitation was a medical stepchild with no alle-
giance. Rehabilitation then was not ready to stand on its own
feet and have an independent position, so physical medicine
'took it under its wing.'"[153] Even the title "physiatrist" was
inaccurate, they claimed, because it only meant "a healer by
physical agents" and "does not include the social, educational, and vocational aspects of rehabilitation, nor does it
include medical care except that given by physical means."[154]
In fact, in the opinion of at least one orthopedic surgeon,
rehabilitation would have developed faster since World
War II if the specialty of physical medicine and rehabilitation
had not been created.[155]

Orthopedists continued their attack on the specialty status
of physical medicine and rehabilitation through the 1960s.
They now claimed that there had not been any growth or
evolution of physiatrists' therapeutic techniques comparable
to those in surgical specialties, internal medicine, or public

health, and that, as a research area, physical medicine was
"sterile" because most questions a physiatrist could investigate were already under investigation by other disciplines.[156]
Some argued that physical medicine and rehabilitation should
be denied recognition as a medical specialty because comprehensive or total medical care in the spirit of physiatry was
the job of every responsible physician.[157] Rehabilitation, in
the eyes of many physicians, was "everybody's business" and
should, at most, develop into a subspecialty of internal medicine. There would then be no function or need for the physiatrist.[158] As a solution to the "problems and limitations of
physical medicine and rehabilitation," orthopedic surgeons
proposed that physiatrists fill a managerial role in medicine.[159]
In this role the physiatrist would become a "super-coordinator
of services without special or unique scientific talents of his
own."[160] However, to do this, wrote one orthopedist, "he
must leave the game of the specialists because the established
rules will not permit him to become a star."[161]

Physiatrists denied charges that physical medicine and rehabilitation was not a legitimate medical specialty. In the mid-
1960s a Commission on Education in Physical Medicine and
Rehabilitation (later changed to the Commission on Rehabilitation Medicine) was formed by the joint efforts of the American Board of Physical Medicine and Rehabilitation and the
American Academy of Physical Medicine and Rehabilitation.
The nine-member commission was to define the basic intellectual structure that set this specialty apart from others, as
well as the "needs which rehabilitation-medicine is uniquely
fitted to fulfill."[162]

Despite organized attempts to define the boundaries of the
specialty, physiatrists continued to be plagued by this problem. The commission, for example, reported in 1968 that when
physiatrists were asked what dissatisfied them about their
specialty, they most commonly pointed to its uncertain status
as a specialty.[163] As one physiatrist exclaimed, "in contrast to
other specialties, it lacks an age, organ, tool, or appendage
to stand on."[164] At the start of the 1980s, even leading physiatrists remained troubled with the question of specialty status, calling their own specialty "difficult" because

the sphere of required knowledge crosses over into almost every specialty and requires frequent interdisciplinary discourse. It may be unpleasant to acknowledge, but it is a delusion to expect medical colleagues . . . to render professional respect when theirs and our pool of knowledge is patently disproportionate.[165]

Moves by occupational and physical therapy to increase autonomy began when physiatry's control over the rehabilitation market was challenged by competing orthopedic surgeons. Physical therapists, in particular, used these squabbles between specialties to court the orthopedic surgeons and to lessen physiatrist influence.[166] Physical therapists could also benefit economically from territorial conflicts between medical specialties by receiving referrals from each group of physicians. To assure continuation of the economically profitable status quo brought on by interspecialty rivalry in the medical profession, physical therapists in the 1970s sought legal protection to work under the general supervision of any physician without a specific prescription.[167]

More significant, allied health workers assumed greater responsibility for the application of rehabilitation treatments as physiatrists abdicated this role.[168] The limited supply of physiatrists in the 1950s and 1960s made it necessary to restrict their clinical responsibilities to diagnosis and supervision of treatment as consultants. Although physical and occupational therapists did not have the same training as physiatrists, they were both cheaper and more plentiful than physicians. Allied health workers were now in a strategic position to take advantage of the demand created for rehabilitation, and in so doing, advance their own autonomy in the division of labor.

By the 1970s physiatrists started to regret the loss of their treatment role—to physical therapists in particular—because the market for them as diagnosticians and consultants was shrinking. As one former president of the congress admitted:

It is no secret that many rehabilitation centers are in financial trouble, and hospital administrators are less sympathetic toward the space and personnel requirements of certain aspects of physical medicine and rehabilitation than they were several years ago. It is apparent that the impetus for expansion is diminishing.[169]

Even physiatrists' traditional stronghold in the VA hospitals weakened as the system retrenched. Symptomatic of their narrowing market, physiatrists decided not to plan physician assistant programs in the 1970s.[170]

Physiatrists bemoaned the fact that "breeds displaying the protective mimicry of physical medicine and rehabilitation flourish in nursing homes and even in hospitals."[171] They now wanted to recapture the commodity they abdicated to therapists and which therapists so willingly assumed. "What should the physiatrist do when the leadership of that allied health group [physical therapy] mounts a misguided, expansive move?" asked one physiatrist. "The answer is simple and painful! Forceful resistance with whatever legitimate means that can be mustered is necessary."[172] Some physiatrists, as well as orthopedic surgeons, started hiring physical therapists in the 1970s as a way of enhancing their own practices and reducing competition from therapists working in the fee-for-service market. Although physical therapists saw such hiring by physicians as preferable to the use of secretaries, office nurses, or "female high school dropouts,"[173] they charged that the decision to hire physical therapists "was made simply because they realized that there was a profit to be made from physical therapy if the therapists were in their employ. The death knell may well be sounding for small, independent practitioners."[174]

Many physiatrists have taken to doing their own physical therapy instead of hiring a therapist or delegating work to someone with less training. "Regretfully, there are physiatrists who never personally rendered a physical treatment, never given a diathermy treatment, or personally directed a gait training or exercise session." Failure to "maintain control of the patient care scene," noted a physiatrist, "leaves a vacuum that the therapist is unwillingly sucked into in the beginning, and then eventually comes to see as his/her proper domain."[175] Some proposals have been made to include a four-to six-month period during the physical medicine residency for specific training in physical therapy equivalent to that received by therapists in certificate programs. This special training "would adequately establish the physiatrists' background and competency in basic tools of the trade. It would not seem too farfetched to award a certificate of competency in physical therapy since comparative educational goals would appear to have been achieved."[176] Some physiatrists are even entering physical therapy schools to qualify as licensed physical therapists.[177] Such a move reduces their competition and makes them eligible for those third-party reimbursements only available to physical therapists.

Physiatrists also sought to maintain control over specific diagnostic techniques that they traditionally performed, but that were increasingly being assumed by other specialists in medicine and by physical therapists. Diagnostic techniques were more than just a way for physiatrists to distinguish their commodity. They were also a way to legitimate their presence in hospitals, to ensure referrals from neighboring specialties such as orthopedics and neurology, and to increase their income.[178] "The wise physiatrist will do tests himself," noted one practitioner, and will offer to support neurological findings whenever possible. "The future of physical medicine depends as much on the diagnostic acumen of physiatrists as their therapeutic ability."[179] Therefore, to secure diagnostic referrals within hospitals, particularly from orthopedics and neurology, "the physical medicine specialist should acquire as much diagnostic equipment as his budget will permit."[180]

The battle for control over diagnostic procedures began when physical therapists, in small numbers, started performing electromyography tests in the 1970s. In 1973 the Section on Physical Medicine and Rehabilitation presented a resolution to the AMA to prohibit the use of electromyography by nonphysicians, and specified that the resolution be distributed by the AMA to all third-party providers as well as individual state licensing boards of medicine and allied health fields.[181] This resolution was amended by the AMA to leave the determination of responsibility for performing electromyography to each state's Board of Medical Examiners.[182]

Electromyography thus was considered by the AMA to be a clinical extension of the physician's examination which should be performed by and/or under the direct supervision of physicians.

At this time the American Board of Physical Medicine and Rehabilitation upgraded its residency requirements in electromyography and electrodiagnosis to further strengthen its position that electromyography required advanced medical training.[183] However, there was no attempt by the academy to preclude any other specialty from incorporating electromyography as part of its residency training. Electromyography, according to the 1975 Academy presidential address, was the same as a laminectomy or a GI examination because they all could be performed by physicians from different specialties.[184]

Physiatrists clearly felt more threatened by physical therapists than by physicians, and focused their attacks on the competency of nonphysicians to perform electromyography. One physician argued that when it came to electromyography, "few without doctoral-level education (academic or medical) can do justice to these patients and to the referring physician." She noted further: "electromyography is a highly subjective skill" that physical therapists do not adequately learn in their training. "The signals are subtle and interpretation depends on a great deal of experience, supported by a firm knowledge of three-dimensional anatomy, neuromuscular physiology, and neuromuscular pathology." Attempts by physical therapists to perform electromyographies, warned this physician, would result in "strong reprisals from those who guard the quality of patient care."[185]

"By what possible authority does she threaten 'reprisal from the guardians of health care?'" questioned one physical therapist. Therapists argued that performing electromyographic tests, measurements, and evaluations was not a highly subjective skill, as argued by physicians, but was a highly technical skill based on a core of knowledge basic to their education. They also disputed the charge made by some physiatrists that they were entering "this sacrosanct territory of physicians in numbers equal to the Mongol hordes that swarmed over

Asia and into Europe in times past."[186] Going on the offensive, another physical therapist commented that M.D. or Ph.D. degrees were not the "*sine qua non* of competent electromyography."[187]

While the APTA moved in 1975 to develop standards for the training of physical therapists in the use of electromyography, not all therapists were pleased with the direction their field was taking. For example, one physical therapist accused her colleagues of being "frustrated physicians" and of "trying to grab the physician's role." She continued: "We are not licensed to diagnose or prescribe. Those therapists who wish this license should get their training in medical school. Our profession should stop confusing 'evaluation' with 'diagnosis' and our schools of physical therapy should stop trying to make physicians of us."[188]

Several angry replies by physical therapists soon appeared in their journal. One asked: "When are we going to stop acting as technicians simply following a prescription without thought?"[189] Another pointed out that physical therapists know more about physical therapy techniques than do physiatrists, as shown by the fact that "many physicians order the *same* treatment for *every* cervical or lumbosacral problem. It is time to become aggressive and not sit back and become 'cookbook' therapists."[190]

As the 1980s began, physical therapy's moves to increase autonomy seemed to indicate a broader definition of the field than that conceived in the 1970s. More than just treating patients without physician prescription or referral, therapists now appeared to be assuming a diagnostic role as well. Recent redefinitions of "physical therapy" supported by the APTA included terms such as "evaluation" and "assessment" and referred to performance and interpretation of tests and measurements to assess pathophysiologic and developmental defects and assist in diagnosis and prognosis. In the opinion of many physiatrists, "that plethora of words is often boundless and ill-defined, yet adds up to activities that mean diagnostic workup and that are well beyond the resources endowed by the professional training of physical therapists."[191] The only way physical therapists could assume such a role, argued physiatrists, would be to expand their training to include "a regime comparable to residency programs."[192]

This is, in fact, what physical therapists are trying to do. In 1979 the APTA decided to require a master's degree as the minimum entry-level education as of 1990.[193] Moreover, at some universities, such as New York University and Marquette, proposals are being made to create a professional doctorate degree in physical therapy which would take six years to complete after high school. Such master's or doctoral programs in physical therapy can then be used to justify the independent practice of therapists even in hospitals, as well as to increase direct third-party reimbursement.[194]

The vogue enjoyed by physical medicine and rehabilitation in the late 1940s and early 1950s passed quickly. The specialty has since been rejected by much of mainstream medicine and absorbed and curtailed by numerous physician and nonphysician groups, most notably orthopedic surgeons and physical therapists. Indeed, physical therapists have questioned whether there is a need to train any more physiatrists, despite manpower predictions by physicians which call for increased production of physiatrists. In attacking these estimates, physical therapists directly challenged the physiatrist's clinical raison d'etre, noting that these projections largely ignored the fact that physical therapists could provide rehabilitation "more efficiently" than physiatrists.[195] What remains of physical medicine and rehabilitation in the 1980s are a few pockets or institutional strongholds where physiatrists retain nominal clinical control over allied health workers, and where allied health workers depend on referrals from physiatrists. By 1980 over 90 percent of referrals to physical therapists came from physicians who were not physiatrists.[196] Without a secure and credible institutional base, the future of physical medicine and rehabilitation as a specialty is dubious.

Epilogue

To accept the natural growth model, we would have to accept that the present structure and domain of rehabilitation medicine could not have been otherwise. But the rehabilitation field could have proceeded along different lines at certain historically critical points. For example, had there not been a war physicians specializing in electrotherapy might never have been accepted into the medical profession. Eventually they might have become direct competitors of physicians, as did osteopaths, chiropractors, and optometrists.

Again, conflicts during World War I between the military and the civilian Federal Board for Vocational Education were crucial in separating the boundaries of medicine and the developing vocational rehabilitation field. This conflict, resolved on the floors of Congress, checked potential medical expansion into rehabilitation, while protecting physician authority from lay interference. Had the surgeon general successfully implemented his plan for comprehensive reconstruction hospitals, present rehabilitation services might be organized along the lines of the mental hospital: a self-contained "therapeutic" community under physician control. Instead, the vocational rehabilitation program developed under the authority of educators, and later under vocational rehabilitation counselors.

Survival of physical therapy physicians also depended on the failure of orthopedic surgeons to construct a system of "orthopedic hospitals" to handle the war wounded. Orthopedic surgeons were unsuccessful because other specialties wanted to be included in this new area of work. The fact that general surgeons thwarted orthopedic surgeons' desires for independence was particularly important because it provided physical therapy physicians with an opportunity during World War II to claim specialty status.[1] Although the AMA gave no indication prior to the war that it would recognize this claim, physical medicine physicians were granted formal specialty status in 1947. Their capacity to incorporate new areas of practice and gain the support of important political allies led to their ascendance in the military and in the Veterans Administration.

The development of allied occupations also does not follow the natural growth model. They entered into subordinate relationships with the medical profession to gain legitimation and the means to structure their labor markets.[2] Without these relationships, physical therapy technicians might have become direct competitors of the physicians performing this work in a manner similar to osteopaths and chiropractors. This would have been unlikely, however, because societal values would have made it difficult for female technicians to compete directly with male physicians. At the least, allied practitioners' private, fee-for-service practice would have been more prevalent than is now the case.

The division of labor among allied occupations also developed and changed through the political activities of occupational associations and the intervention of external sources of authority. For example, successful efforts by physical therapists to restrict the markets of corrective therapists helped establish the former as the most utilized therapists in rehabilitation.[3] The conflict during World War II between physical and occupational therapists over responsibility for amputee rehabilitation resulted in the demarcation of their boundaries. The surgeon general authorized physical therapists to handle lower extremity amputees, while occupational therapists were to work only with upper extremity cases.[4] In short, these critical incidents demonstrate that the current rehabilitation division of labor might have developed differently.

The Bases for Rigidity and Imperialism

Although the division of labor depends on the interplay of the marketplace and history, it is clear that occupations are not inherently imperialistic: they are often inflexible and they often fail to take advantage of opportunities to expand their markets. If they were inherently imperialistic, newcomers would have little chance to organize for the purpose of claiming a new area of work. In rehabilitation, however, new occupations formed, at least in part, because of the rigidity of existing groups of workers. It is important to understand why this rigidity occurs because it is as much a force in shaping the division of labor as is occupational imperialism.

Occupational rigidity results from the failure to balance two different, and at times opposing, requirements for group survival. The first requirement is to remain open to new opportunities for expansion. Developing occupations must be willing to revise their cognitive bases, suspend interest in status mobility, and absorb and expand into new areas of work. The second requirement is to secure territory already gained. Developing occupations must define the boundaries of their knowledge, raise entry standards to increase social status, and pursue exclusive market controls.

These two requirements can pose dilemmas. Cognitive closure, for example, can interfere with the need to remain open to new possibilities for expansion. If workers share a specific body of knowledge, they are likely to develop a common framework for interpreting the external world. Within this framework they may not perceive potential opportunities or may consider them unrelated to their work. If a group fails to perceive new areas of practice, it will be unable to expand its services and markets, thus bringing the requirement to delimit the cognitive base into conflict with further development and control of the marketplace.

Similarly, the pursuit of social status usually supports market interests, but it also can impede market expansion and control. Establishing the definitive nature of a commodity involves developing and enforcing standards for group membership. Status mobility depends on the constant raising of standards, accomplished by eliminating dirty work and requiring longer training in increasingly complex knowledge. Barriers to expansion occur when status interests lead the group to reject new markets because these require lower levels of skill than are currently used. The result is that a new, potentially competitive occupation may form.

Finally, exclusive market controls also result in rigidities. The task is to structure the labor market by guaranteeing demand for services which only one group can provide. The capacity to control occupational entry in combination with a defined and guaranteed demand constitutes market control. Once market closure is achieved, the group attempts to raise its standards by increasing minimal requirements for entry and employment. This serves, however, to inhibit the ability to respond to new opportunities. Most important, the standards regulating entry make it difficult to increase worker supply to meet rising demand, especially during wartime, and open the way for the formation of a new occupation.

In the rehabilitation field, we saw the formation of new occupations because of the rapid increase in wartime demand and the failure of existing groups to meet that demand. For example, the status concerns and work conception of nurses during World War I caused a lack of interest in rehabilitation. This new area of work was seen as a potential threat to their professionalizing activities and "cherished standards"; they expressed concern about blurring the line they established between the "nurse" and the "untrained" person.[5] This goal of excluding the untrained to delimit occupational boundaries and raise status led nurses to reject this new work and provided an opportunity for physical therapy to develop after the war.

The creation in the late 1940s of a rehabilitation nursing specialty indicates that nurses then wanted to be involved in rehabilitative work. The unanswerable question is whether physical therapy would have emerged if nurses incorporated this work. Another possibility would have been for nurses to handle this work during the war, and later spin off a specialized segment to form a new occupation. If this had occurred, it is likely that the conception of their work and their position in the division of labor would have been different from that of physical therapists.

The formation of corrective therapy during World War II can also be traced to an existing group's failure to meet the demand for assistance in physical rehabilitation of the war wounded. In this instance, the physical therapists' status concerns and work conception were less important than their inability to supply enough workers to meet demand. During the war physical therapists were concerned about their standards and position in civilian and military markets. While they reduced their standards to some extent, it was impossible to train enough workers, even with a shortened training period. As a result, a new occupation developed which performed tasks similar to those of the physical therapist. After the war these individuals organized and eventually became known as corrective therapists.

Failure to provide an adequate worker supply can be problematic in peacetime as well as wartime. The need to keep supply in line with demand is a continuing issue for allied occupations. Like craft occupations, allied groups had to meet a rising demand resulting, in part, from pressure they put on institutions to employ only certified or licensed individuals. Unless a group can produce enough workers, gains made by creating a guaranteed demand will be negated through the hiring of less trained and cheaper workers. Pursuit of exclusive control over entry and standards, therefore, can impede market closure. When the group's material rewards are relatively low, high entry costs make it difficult to recruit workers. Since this provides opportunities for new occupations to develop, it represents an ongoing dynamic favoring further specialization.

Recruiting members has been especially problematic for rehabilitation medicine physicians. As a marginal group in the medical profession, they attempted to convince other physicians that their methods were useful. This strategy, however, prevented them from establishing closure around a specific area of claimed expertise and made it difficult to persuade other physicians that their specialty had value.

Groups may try to balance the two opposing requirements for occupational survival through ideological means. For the most part, the pre-World War I electrotherapeutists did not try to establish a claim to unique expertise, but instead emphasized the general utility of their techniques; thus, the need to gain acceptance and establish themselves in referral networks prevented cognitive closure. After the war the marginal status of these physicians and the AMA's antagonism toward specialization continued to hinder any claim of special expertise. Until the early 1930s, they conceptualized their methods as a third modality of medicine, in addition to drugs and surgery. Their need to gain acceptance and potential recruits still prevented the firm delimitation of the group's boundaries.

When the AMA eventually recognized specialties, physical medicine physicians altered their conceptions and strategies. They developed a "bridging" ideology, stating that all physicians could perform simple procedures, while difficult cases demanded special expertise. In the 1940s they increasingly stressed a specialized expertise rooted in physics, which uniquely enabled them to diagnose and manage the "third stage" of illness. Their improved postwar position provided the opportunity to develop a new conception of their work and a new ideology to legitimate their existence as a specialty.

The conflict between the two requirements may also be resolved organizationally. Physiatrists formed a separate organization, known today as the American Academy of Physical Medicine and Rehabilitation, that would be open only to physicians who specialized in physical therapy for at least five years and who were in teaching or leadership positions. This association provided an exclusive domain, and later became the mechanism for defining specialty membership. The original organization, currently named the American Congress of Rehabilitation Medicine, continues to crusade for acceptance and converts. As a result of a wider audience (due to increased government subsidization), the congress opened itself in recent years to any interested "professional" working in the rehabilitation field.[6]

Our work also shows that occupations will be imperialistic under certain conditions. In the nineteenth century, the rise of "scientific" medicine and the availability of scientifically derived technologies led medical segments to incorporate areas of practice or techniques which could be connected to modern science. We saw, for example, how the American Electro-Therapeutic Association and the homeopathic National Society of Electro-Therapeutics claimed electrical devices and sought to establish the efficacy of these techniques. Similarly, they claimed the newly discovered x-ray in the 1890s, as did other groups that organized around this device. Even during this highly imperialistic period, however, the tendency of electrotherapeutists toward paradigmatic exclusiveness (the emphasis on electrical devices) resulted in their giving only secondary importance to the x-ray, which eventually became the sole purview of the segment that originally organized around it. Occupational imperialism, then, is related to a competitive economic situation and to group perceptions about whether a new area of practice will promote its intellectual and material interests.

The rigidification of the medical market in the twentieth century has been unfavorable to medical imperialism. Despite this, two factors encouraged occupations to expand. First, marginal status favored a flexible posture vis-à-vis new opportunities. Marginal groups, for example, could react to wartime demands because they wanted to increase their numbers; thus, both physical medicine physicians and occupational therapists have been able to redirect their focus during wartime. Second, occupations are more likely to claim an area of practice, even a previously ignored one, when an existing competitor tries to establish exclusive control. This can be seen in the way physical therapists reacted when corrective therapists claimed exercise as part of their unique expertise.

For the most part, however, twentieth-century social and market contexts have discouraged imperialism. Recently this situation has changed, in part because occupations realized that earlier failures to incorporate new areas of practice facilitated the development of competing groups, but principally because a more competitive economic market was created by the federal government in the 1960s and 1970s. The imperialistic posture of allied occupations was a clear response to this enlarged federal role. By guaranteeing demand for services previously ignored by the fee-for-service market, especially for the disabled and chronically ill, federal programs opened new markets outside the medical profession's control. These new opportunities encouraged political awareness by allied occupations, which was manifested in renewed interest in state licensing, struggle over accreditation of educational institutions, creation of affiliations with public and private organizations that influence health-related institutions, and, especially, lobbying efforts to gain favorable consideration in federal legislation and programs.

By creating new markets and demand for rehabilitation services, the federal government stimulated the number of competitors in the rehabilitation field and created pressure for cheaper labor sources. In response, physical and occupational therapy have formalized assistant levels.[7] In meeting the demand for lesser skilled workers by diverting their unwanted work to insiders under their control, allied groups eliminate one of the causes of specialization. They can push for higher levels of educational requirements and delegate lower-level tasks without providing the opportunity for a new occupation to develop. Similarly, it is possible to claim areas of practice low in status, since these can be delegated to assistants.

This phenomenon of internal specialization indicates that allied groups are less concerned about internal homogeneity, necessary for occupational unification and closure, than about the proliferation of potential competitors. If internal segments can be prevented from spinning off, the proliferation of new occupations can be resisted. These internal segments will then create "mini-domains," within which they can control the content of work. There is a delicate balance, however, between the need to maintain internal cohesion and the need to recognize special interests within an occupation. If these interest groups are not recognized by formal titles or structural differentiation, they may attempt to separate from the parent group and develop their own independent identity; yet, a high degree of internal specialization may threaten group cohesiveness and provide the basis for the later separation into segments. The ideal for the parent organization appears to be recognition of specialized interests, but a minimizing of the role and strength of the subunits formed on the basis of these interests.

Contrary to the notion that an occupation focuses on status mobility once it is established in the market,[8] rehabilitation groups are more concerned than ever with extending and controlling markets. Although the federal government has been the source of this activity, it failed to direct development of these new markets even before the current emphasis on deregulation. One notable example was the founding, in 1967, of the American Society of Allied Health Professions. Funded by the Allied Health Act of 1966, ASAHP was formed in response to complaints by educational institutions and the federal government about fragmentation of the health system. The society became involved in the controversial areas of accreditation and certification, and widened its base to include the allied occupations and representatives of educational institutions. It sought to provide a single voice for the allied groups and a mechanism for overcoming occupational specialization in favor of more generalized approaches to education and practice.

Although the AOTA and APTA hoped that the ASAHP would become a counterbalance to the medical profession by strengthening the identity, independence, and alliances of allied health occupations, both organizations quit ASAHP in the early 1970s. Physical and occupational therapists resented the fact that those ASAHP members who spoke for the society and determined its policy were predominantly physicians.[9] In particular, therapists opposed attempts by physicians to homogenize the allied health occupations through ASAHP. One physical therapist called ASAHP a "Dean's Club," which took the allied health occupations "out of the frying pan and into the fire."[10] Although physical therapy rejoined the society, current APTA officials conclude that it has little impact because it has been unable to overcome specialized occupational interests.[11]

Government officials expressed concern in the early 1970s over fragmentation, but were no more successful than the ASAHP in halting it. This concern was manifested in a 1971 call, made jointly by the federal government, the AMA, and the AHA, for a voluntary two-year moratorium on licensing of allied health occupations.[12] Although the moratorium was presented as a way to prevent further fragmentation of the existing system of health manpower, it was not an expression of real concern with the basic causes of fragmentation. The roots of fragmentation lie more in the internal specialization of the medical profession than in the continued specialization of allied health occupations. The moratorium reflected the desire of major institutions to maintain control over the health care system; it was not an attempt to overcome a system of fragmented patient care, but an effort to reestablish control over workers and the labor process involved in the production of health services.

This desire to regain control over allied health workers was reflected in a report, issued in 1973, calling for a two-year extension of the original moratorium. The stated purpose of the moratorium, according to this report, was to provide time to study the licensure issue and to develop criteria to determine which occupations should be licensed. Unlicensed allied occupations, however, saw the moratorium as an attempt to limit their autonomy and criticized the government for this. The authors of the 1973 report defended their position by saying that the initiative did not come from the government but rather from the AMA and AHA, and by rejecting criticisms that it was a stopgap or holding action: "it was not intended as a call for inaction or for simply maintaining the *status quo* of licensed versus unlicensed health occupations."[13]

The AMA's concern over fragmentation must be understood as a response to the threat of greater economic competition and loss of control over allied health occupations. This resulted in its joining forces with the federal government and the AHA to block further licensing through the imposition of a moratorium, thereby furthering its long-standing policy of opposition to the licensing of allied health occupations.[14] The real issue for the medical profession is the maintenance of its monopolistic privileges in the face of a rebellion by allied health occupations.

The federal government and other groups, such as hospital administrators and public health agencies, also have an interest in controlling allied health occupations. Rather than wanting to prevent further specialization, as their support for the licensing moratorium suggested, these groups are really concerned with establishing a more "rational" system of health care.[15] Their concern has not led, however, to a direct attack on the ultimate basis of occupational control of work: the medical profession's legal authority to achieve a monopoly of the market for health care services. Confrontation with the power of organized medicine is thereby avoided; the dominant interests can continue to pursue their own goals within a system maintained by their symbiotic relationship.[16]

It cannot be assumed that the government, through special agencies, can prevent further fragmentation, let alone reverse that which exists. The Veterans Administration's attempt to merge occupations is instructive. Although situated in the VA, occupations successfully resisted administrative authority. Once organized, these groups have a great capacity for survival. (Since the war no occupation in rehabilitation has surrendered its independence.) If the VA could not control groups that developed within it, then other federal agencies will probably have little effect on occupations whose authority is rooted outside the federal bureaucracy. Given the government's failure to direct the organization of work, the future division of labor in rehabilitation will be shaped largely by struggles among occupations to improve their market position.

Appendixes

Appendix A

CHANGES IN OCCUPATIONAL TITLES

	1890–1917	1917–1920	1920–1941	1941–1950
Physicians:	electrotherapeutists	physiotherapists	physical therapy physicians	physiatrists
Allied Workers:		reconstruction aides	physiotherapists, physiotherapy technicians, physical therapy technicians	physical therapists
		reconstruction aides	occupational therapists	

Appendix B

PROFESSIONAL ASSOCIATIONS AND JOURNALS: PHYSICIANS

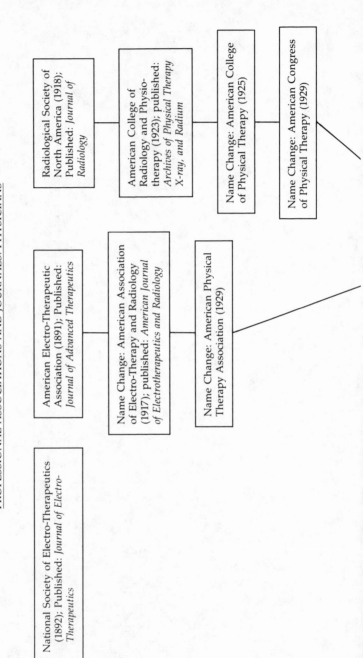

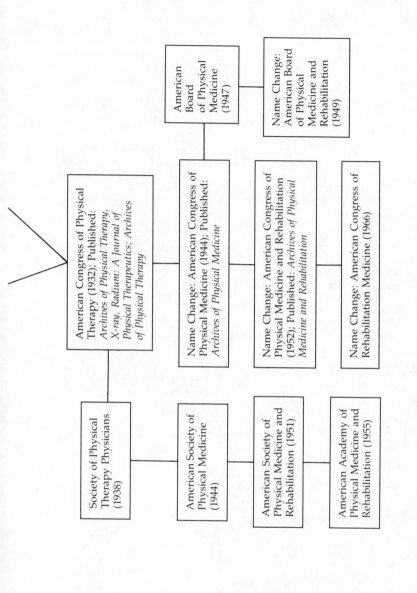

American Congress of Physical Therapy (1932); Published: *Archives of Physical Therapy, X-ray, Radium: A Journal of Physical Therapeutics; Archives of Physical Therapy*

Name Change: American Congress of Physical Medicine (1944); Published: *Archives of Physical Medicine*

Name Change: American Congress of Physical Medicine and Rehabilitation (1952); Published: *Archives of Physical Medicine and Rehabilitation*

Name Change: American Congress of Rehabilitation Medicine (1966)

American Board of Physical Medicine (1947)

Name Change: American Board of Physical Medicine and Rehabilitation (1949)

Society of Physical Therapy Physicians (1938)

American Society of Physical Medicine (1944)

American Society of Physical Medicine and Rehabilitation (1951)

American Academy of Physical Medicine and Rehabilitation (1955)

Appendix C

PROFESSIONAL ASSOCIATIONS AND
JOURNALS: ALLIED OCCUPATIONS

National Society for the
Promotion of Occupational
Therapy (1917); Published:
Maryland Psychiatric Quarterly

American Women's Physical
Therapeutical Association
(1921)

Name Change: American
Occupational Therapy
Association (1923); Published:
*Occupational Therapy and
Rehabilitation; American Journal of
Occupational Therapy*

Name Change: American
Physiotherapy Association
(1922); Published: *Physiotherapy
Review; Physical Therapy Review*

Name Change: American
Physical Therapy Association
(1946); Published: *Journal of
the American Physical Therapy
Association; Physical Therapy*

Notes

1. Introduction

1. Richard M. Magraw, *Ferment in Medicine* (Philadelphia: W. B. Saunders Company, 1969), p. 149.

2. Harold M. Goldstein and Morris A. Horowitz, *Entry-Level Health Occupations: Development and Future* (Baltimore: The Johns Hopkins University Press, 1971), pp. 5–6.

3. Eliot Freidson, "Professions and the Occupational Principle," in *The Professions and Their Prospects,* ed. Eliot Freidson (Beverly Hills: Sage Publications, 1973), p. 24.

4. June S. Rothberg, "Territorial Imperatives and the Boundaries of Professional Practice in Rehabilitation," *Archives of Physical Medicine and Rehabilitation* 52 (1971): 397.

5. Stanley Joel Reiser, *Medicine and the Reign of Technology* (Cambridge: Cambridge University Press, 1978), p. 146.

6. Magraw, *Ferment in Medicine,* p. 149.

7. E. L. Stebbins, "Why This Conference?" *Journal of the American Medical Association* 170 (1959): 284–285.

8. Charles A. Beard, "Introduction," in J. B. Bury, *The Idea of Progress: An Inquiry Into Its Origin and Growth* (New York: Dover Publications, 1960), pp. ix-xl.

9. Kenneth Bock, *Human Nature and History: A Response to Sociobiology* (New York: Columbia University Press, 1980); and Frederick J. Teggart, *Theory of History* (New Haven: Yale University Press, 1925).

10. Robert Nisbet, *Social Change and History: Aspects of the Western Theory of Development* (London: Oxford University Press, 1969).

11. Adam Smith, *An Inquiry Into the Nature and Causes of the Wealth of Nations* (New York: Random House, 1937), chaps. 1, 3; and Herbert Spencer, *Principles of Sociology, Vol. III* (New York: D. Appleton and Company, 1914), pts. VII–VIII.

178   NOTES TO PAGES 4–13

12. Eliot Freidson, "The Division of Labor as Social Interaction," *Social Problems* 23 (1976): 304–313.

13. Émile Durkheim, *The Division of Labor in Society* (New York: The Macmillan Company, 1933).

14. Theodore Kemper, "The Division of Labor: A Post-Durkheimian Analytical View," *American Sociological Review* 37 (1972): 739–741.

15. William Goode, "Encroachment, Charlatanism, and the Emerging Profession: Psychology, Sociology, and Medicine," *American Sociological Review* 25 (1960): 902–914.

16. William Goode, "Theoretical Limits of Professionalization," in *The Semi-Professions and Their Organization*, ed. A. Etzioni (New York: The Free Press, 1969), pp. 266–313.

17. Thomas Kuhn, *The Structure of Scientific Revolutions* (Chicago: The University of Chicago Press, 1970).

18. Georges Sorel, *The Illusions of Progress* (Berkeley: University of California Press, 1969).

19. Nisbet, *Social Change and History*, pp. 249–250.

20. Iago Galdston, "The Birth and Death of Specialties," *Journal of the American Medical Association* 167 (1958): 2056; Elizabeth Garnsey, "The Rediscovery of the Division of Labor," *Theory and Society* 10 (1981) 337; and Elliott Krause, *Division of Labor: A Political Perspective* (Westport, Conn.: Greenwood Press, 1982).

21. See, e.g., Jeffrey Berlant, *Profession and Monopoly* (Berkeley, Los Angeles, London: University of California Press, 1975); Carol Brown, "The Division of Laborers: Allied Health Professions," *International Journal of Health Services* 3 (1973): 435–445; E. Richard Brown, *Rockefeller Medicine Men* (Berkeley, Los Angeles, London: University of California Press, 1979); Carol L. Kronus, "The Evolution of Occupational Power," *Sociology of Work and Occupations* 3 (1976): 3–38; and William D. White, *Public Health and Private Gain* (Chicago: Maaroufa Press, 1979).

22. Magali Sarfatti Larson, *The Rise of Professionalism: A Sociological Analysis* (Berkeley, Los Angeles, London: University of California Press, 1977).

23. Glenn Gritzer, "Occupational Specialization in Medicine: Knowledge and Market Explanations," in *Research in the Sociology of Health Care*, vol. 2, ed. Julius A. Roth (Greenwich, Conn.: JAI Press, 1982), pp. 251–283.

24. Rothberg, "Territorial Imperatives and the Boundaries of Professional Practice in Rehabilitation," pp. 397–412.

25. Ibid., p. 397.

26. Frank H. Krusen, "Historical Development in Physical Medicine and Rehabilitation During the Last Forty Years," *Archives of Physical Medicine and Rehabilitation* 50 (1969): 1–5.

27. Frank H. Krusen, "History and Development of Physical Medicine," in *Physical Medicine in General Practice*, ed. Arthur L. Watkins (Philadelphia: J. B. Lippincott, 1946), pp. 5, 8.

2: The Bases for Specialization, 1890–1917

1. Sidney Licht, "History of Electrotherapy," in *Therapeutic Electricity and Ultraviolet Radiation*, ed. Sidney Licht (Baltimore: Waverly Press, 1959), pp. 5–6.

2. Benjamin Franklin, "An Account of the Effects of Electricity in Paralytic Cases," *Philosophical Transactions* 50 (1759): 481.

3. Licht, "History of Electrotherapy," p. 15.

4. Fielding Garrison, *An Introduction to the History of Medicine* (Philadelphia: W. B. Saunders Co., 1914), p. 328.

5. Licht, "History of Electrotherapy," p. 17.

6. T. Gale, *Electricity or Ethereal Fire. Theory and Practice of Medical Electricity* (Troy, N.Y.: Moffitt and Lyons, 1802), pp. 6, 99, 242.

7. *Boston Medical and Surgical Journal* 31 (December 25, 1844): 424–425.

8. "Electricity as a Remedy in Nervous Diseases," *Boston Medical and Surgical Journal* 61 (August 4, 1859): 14.

9. Licht, "History of Electrotherapy," p. 19.

10. A. C. Garratt, *Electro-Physiology and Electro-Therapeutics: Showing the Best Methods for the Medical Uses of Electricity* (Boston, 1860).

11. Licht, "History of Electrotherapy," p. 19.

12. George Beard and A. D. Rockwell, *A Practical Treatise on the Medical and Surgical Uses of Electricity* (New York: William Wood and Co., 1867), p. 11.

13. Review of *Medical and Surgical Uses of Electricity*, 3d ed., by George Beard and A. D. Rockwell, *Philadelphia Medical Times* 5 (February 27, 1875): 348–349.

14. *American Journal of Electrology and Neurology* 1 (July 1, 1879): 69.

15. John S. Haller, *American Medicine in Transition 1840–1910* (Urbana: University of Illinois Press, 1981), pp. 174–191.

16. Harold Speert, *Obstetrics and Gynecology in America: A History* (Chicago: American College of Obstetricians and Gynecologists, 1980), p. 60.

17. Ibid., p. 63.

18. William Harvey King, *History of Homeopathy* (New York: The Lewis Publishing Co., 1905), pp. 347–348.

19. William Harvey King, *Electro-Therapeutics or Electricity in its Relation to Medicine and Surgery* (New York: A. L. Chatterton and Co., 1889).

20. "Historical Memoranda," *Transactions of the American Electro-Therapeutic Association* 2 (1892): 13.

21. *Journal of Electro-Therapeutics* 10 (1892): 230–231.

22. *Journal of Electro-Therapeutics* 14 (1896): 230–239.

23. W. J. Morton, "Opening Comments," *Transactions of the American Electro-Therapeutic Association* 2 (1892): 3–4.

24. *Transactions of the American Electro-Therapeutic Association* 2 (1892): 1.

25. M. C. F. Love, "Some Opinions on the Use of Electricity in Gynecology," *Journal of Electro-Therapeutics* 8 (June 1890): 83.

26. *JAMA* 26 (1896): 446, 1361, 1896.

27. *Journal of Electro-Therapeutics* 11 (1893): 45.

28. William L. Jackson, "The Development of Electro-Therapeutics and Its Relation to the Practice of Medicine," *Journal of Electro-Therapeutics* 13 (1895): 223.

29. "Will it Pay?" *Journal of Electro-Therapeutics* 18 (1900): 34–35.

30. *Journal of Electro-Therapeutics* 10 (1892): 231.

31. William Harvey King, "The Necessary Requirements to Practice Electro-Therapeutics," *Journal of Electro-Therapeutics* 8 (1890): 184.

32. *Journal of Electro-Therapeutics* 11 (1893): 45.

33. *JAMA* 26 (1896): 446, 1361.

34. *Transactions of the American Electro-Therapeutic Association* 9 (1899).

35. "The Electro-Therapist as a Specialist," *Journal of Electro-Therapeutics* 14 (1896): 239–248.

36. Frank Gardner, "Presidential Address," *Journal of Electro-Therapeutics* 16 (1898): 13.

37. "Some of the Causes Which Retard the More Rapid Progress of Electro-Therapeutics," *Journal of Electro-Therapeutics* 10 (1892): 65.

38. *Journal of Electro-Therapeutics* 8 (1890): 117, 184, 1890; ibid. 9 (1891): 41–42.

39. William Harvey King, "Quackery and Electro-Therapeutics," *Journal of Electro-Therapeutics* 10 (1892): 42.

40. H. C. Bennett, "Electric Massage and Vibration," *The Electro-Therapeutist* 4 (1900): 51–56.

41. King, "Quackery and Electro-Therapeutics," pp. 41–45.

42. Jackson, "The Development of Electro-Therapeutics and Its Relation to the Practice of Medicine," p. 223.

43. Hills Cole, "The Use of Electricity in General Medicine," *Journal of Electro-Therapeutics* 16 (1898): 183.

44. Gardner, "Presidential Address," pp. 11–12.

45. Jackson, "The Development of Electro-Therapeutics and Its Relation to the Practice of Medicine," pp. 223–224.

46. F. Morse, "Our Association," *Journal of Advanced Therapeutics* 20 (1902): 637.

47. A. D. Rockwell, "The General Therapeutical Action of Electricity," *Journal of Electro-Therapeutics* 8 (1890): 3–6.

48. S. H. Monell, *Electricity in Health and Disease* (New York: McGraw Publishing Co., 1907), p. 319; Mihran Krikor Kassabian, *Roentgen Rays and Electro-Therapeutics* (Philadelphia: J. B. Lippincott, 1907), p. xxxi.

49. *Transactions of the American Electro-Therapeutic Association* 6 (1896): 26.

50. Spectator, "Letter from Paris," *Boston Medical and Surgical Journal* 157 (December 5, 1907): 778.

51. Ibid.

52. "Dr. William Benham Snow," *Physical Therapeutics* 49 (1931): 44–46; William L. Clark, "An Appreciation of the Life and Work of Dr. William Benham Snow," *Physical Therapeutics* 49 (1931): 330–336.

53. *Journal of Advanced Therapeutics* 24 (1906): 32.

54. "Physical Therapeutics," *Journal of Advanced Therapeutics* 20 (1902): 43–44.

55. Ibid.

56. J. A. Riviere, "Physicotherapy of Neurasthenia," *Journal of Advanced Therapeutics* 23 (1905): 319–326.

57. *Journal of Advanced Therapeutics* 22 (1904): 134–135.

58. "A Change in Name for the American Electro-Therapeutic Association," *Journal of Advanced Therapeutics* 24 (1906) 466–467.

59. "Association of Physical Methods," *Journal of Advanced Therapeutics* 22 (1904): 490.

60. William Harvey King, "The Roentgen Rays," *Journal of Electro-Therapeutics* 14 (1896): 124–125.

61. S. H. Monell, "The Advisability of X-rays," *American X-Ray Journal* 1 (1897): 96–97.

62. F. Kolle, "Roentgenogram Ethics," *American X-Ray Journal* 2 (1898): 210–211.

63. Glenn Gritzer, "Occupational Specialization in Medicine: Knowledge and Market Explanations," in *Research in the Sociology of Health Care*, vol. 2, ed. Julius A. Roth (Greenwich, Conn.: JAI Press, 1982).

64. *Journal of Electro-Therapeutics* 15 (1897): 208; ibid. 18 (1900): 314.

65. *Journal of Advanced Therapeutics* 20 (1902): 702.

66. *Journal of Advanced Therapeutics* 22 (1904): 22.

67. "The Twelfth Annual Meeting of the American Electro-Therapeutic Association," *Journal of Advanced Therapeutics* 20 (1902): 667.

68. *Journal of Electro-Therapeutics* 15 (1897): 62.

69. Edward Skinner, "The Organization of the Roentgen Society of the United States Documentary Evidence and Comment," in *The American Roentgen Ray Society, 1900–1950* (Springfield, Ill.: Charles C Thomas, 1950), pp. 5–14.

70. Charles O. Files, "Some Obstacles to the Progress of Electro-Therapeutics," *Journal of Advanced Therapeutics* 21 (1903): 402.

71. "Therapeutic Discrimination," *Journal of Advanced Therapeutics* 20 (1902): 117; "Physical Methods Will Replace Many Surgical Procedures in the Future," ibid., p. 522; "Recognition of the X-Ray in the Treatment of Malignant Diseases," ibid., p. 585.

72. "Want of Professional Knowledge Upon Important Subjects," *Journal of Advanced Therapeutics* 20 (1902): 319.

73. "Medical Electricity," *Journal of Advanced Therapeutics* 20 (1902): 394; "Science vs. Empiricism in Electro-Therapeutics," ibid. 31 (1913): 307.

74. "The Notion that Electro-Therapeutics in Medicine Is Essentially Psychic," *American Journal of Electro-Therapeutics and Radiology* 35 (1917): 228.

75. "The Attitude of the Neurologists towards Physical Therapeutics," *Journal of Advanced Therapeutics* 26 (1908): 460–461; "A Physical Basis for Most Cases of Functional Disorder," ibid., pp. 575–576.

76. *Journal of Advanced Therapeutics* 22 (1904): 692.

77. "Proposal for a Subdivision of the Fourth Section (Section on Therapeutics) of the International Medical Congress into Three Branches," *Journal of Advanced Therapeutics* 24 (1906): 199.

78. "Recognition of Electro-Therapeutics by the Medical Profession," *Journal of Advanced Therapeutics* 25 (1907): 195–196; "A Section of Physical Therapeutics for the American Medical Association," ibid., p. 254.

79. John T. Rankin, "Manual Therapy, An Invaluable Aid to the Electro-Therapeutist—A Plea for Its General Adoption," *Journal of Advanced Therapeutics* 24 (1906): 66–67.

80. Ibid., p. 68.

81. *JAMA* 26 (March 21, 1896): 587.

82. "Misconceptions Concerning Effects of Electro-Therapeutic Apparatus," *Journal of Advanced Therapeutics* 24 (1906): 137; "The Law and the Medical Profession," ibid., pp. 465–466.

83. "Why Are Static Machines So Much in Disuse?" *Journal of Advanced Therapeutics* 28 (1910): 317.

84. Francis Howard Humphris, "Presidential Address," *Journal of Advanced Therapeutics* 31 (1913): 349.

85. J. C. Walton, "Is the Present Attitude of the Medical Profession Towards Physical Therapeutics Justifiable?" *Journal of Advanced Therapeutics* 30 (1912): 143–157.

86. "The Attitude of the Profession Towards Physicians Who Employ Physical Therapeutics and How to Meet It," *Journal of Advanced Therapeutics* 28 (1910): 415.

87. Anthony Bassler, "Some Ideas Pertaining to Electro-Therapeutics," *Journal of Advanced Therapeutics* 31 (1913): 445.

88. "Signs of Awakening of the Editor of the Official Organ of the American Medical Association," *Journal of Advanced Therapeutics* 31 (1913): 222–223; "The Attitude of the Profession Towards Physicians Who Employ Physical Therapeutics and How to Meet It," ibid., p. 415.

89. "The Modern Status of Medical Science," *Journal of Advanced Therapeutics* 31 (1913): 307–309.

90. "The American Journal of Electro-Therapeutics and Radiology," *Journal of Advanced Therapeutics* 33 (1915): 473–474.

91. "The Specialist Versus the General Practitioner," *American Journal of Electro-Therapeutics and Radiology* 34 (1916): 546.

92. "The Scope and Utility of the Roentgen Examination," *American Journal of Electro-Therapeutics and Radiology* 35 (1917): 32.

93. The Unscientific Conception of the Monotherapist," *American Journal of Electro-Therapeutics and Radiology* 35 (1917): 138–139.

94. "The Specialist Versus the General Practitioner," p. 547.
95. *Journal of Advanced Therapeutics* 34 (1916): 57–58.
96. "The Specialist Versus the General Practitioner," p. 547.

3: War and the Organization of Work, 1917-1920

1. Alexander Lambert, "Medicine, A Determining Factor in War," *JAMA* 72 (1919): 1721.
2. "Compulsory Health Insurance," *JAMA* 68 (1917): 292; "Underlying Principles of Workmen's Compensation Laws," ibid., pp. 1822–1823.
3. Quoted in the *Joint Committee on Education and Labor, April 30–May 2, 1918* (S.4284, H.R. 11367, 65th Congress, 2d Session), p. 149.
4. Harry Mock, "Industrial Medicine and Surgery: The New Specialty," *JAMA* 68 (1917): 1.
5. "Reconstruction and Rehabilitation of Disabled Soldiers," *JAMA* 70 (1918): 1924.
6. "Industrial Medicine in the Placement of Returned Soldiers," *JAMA* 71 (1918): 1829–1830.
7. A. M. Phelps, "Presidential Address," *Transactions of the American Orthopedic Association* 7 (1894): 31–42.
8. W. DeForest, "Presidential Address," *Transactions of the American Orthopedic Association* 3 (1890): 2; V. P. Gibney, "Orthopedic Surgery: Its Definition and Scope," ibid. 4 (1891): 326–338.
9. Phelps, "Presidential Address," pp. 31–42: A. J. Steele, "The Orthopedic Work of the Late Mr. Thomas," *Transactions of the American Orthopedic Association* 4 (1891): 4–12.
10. "Report of Committee on Orthopedic Preparedness," *Transactions of the Section on Orthopedic Surgery,* 1917, pp. 253–254.
11. *The Medical Department of the U.S. Army in the World War* (Washington, D.C.: U.S. Government Printing Office, 1923), I: 425.
12. Ibid., p. 426.
13. Ibid., pp. 406–408.
14. C. Herman Bucholz, "Six Years Experience at the Medico-mechanical Department of the Massachusetts General Hospital," *JAMA* 63 (1914): 1733.
15. Nathaniel Allison, "Orthopedic Surgery and the Crippled," *JAMA* 65 (1915): 753–754.
16. "Joel E. Goldthwait," *Harvard Medical Alumni Bulletin* 35 (Spring 1961): 64.
17. "Elliott Gray Brackett, 1860–1942," *Harvard Medical Alumni Bulletin* 17 (April 1943): 63–64.
18. Robert Osgood, "Orthopedic Surgery in War Time," *JAMA* 67 (1916): 420.

19. Joel E. Goldthwait, "The Orthopedic Preparedness of the Nation," *American Journal of Orthopedic Surgery* 15 (1917): 219–220.

20. "Meeting of the Boston Orthopedic Club at the Boston Medical Library, Saturday Evening, October 6, 1917," *American Journal of Orthopedic Surgery* 15 (1917): 848.

21. John Porter, "Orthopedic Surgery and the War," *American Journal of Orthopedic Surgery* 16 (1918): 414.

22. "The Scope of a Reconstruction Hospital," *American Journal of Orthopedic Surgery* 15 (1917): 609.

23. "Report of Committee on Orthopedic Preparedness," pp. 248–249; and Joel E. Goldthwait, "Organization of the Division of Orthopedic Surgery in the U.S. Army with the Expeditionary Force," *American Journal of Orthopedic Surgery* 16 (1918): 288.

24. Joel E. Goldthwait, "The Place of Orthopedic Surgery in War," *American Journal of Orthopedic Surgery* 15 (1917): 679–680; and "Reconstruction," ibid., p. 545.

25. Osgood, "Orthopedic Surgery in War Time," p. 418.

26. "The Function of Orthopedic Surgery in the War," *JAMA* 69 (1917): 2123.

27. "Report of Committee on Orthopedic Preparedness," p. 248.

28. "The Function of Orthopedic Surgery in the War," p. 2123.

29. *The Medical Department of the U.S. Army in the World War* XIII: 4.

30. "Meeting of the Boston Orthopedic Club at the Boston Medical Library, Saturday Evening, October 6, 1917," p. 851.

31. Ibid., p. 854.

32. *The Medical Department of the U.S. Army in the World War* I: 474.

33. *The Medical Department of the U.S. Army in the World War* XI: 551.

34. *The Medical Department of the U.S. Army in the World War* I: 429–431.

35. Ibid., pp. 432–434.

36. Ibid., pp. 431–432.

37. *JAMA* 70 (1918): 928.

38. *The Medical Department of the U.S. Army in the World War* I: 476.

39. *American Journal of Electro-Therapeutics and Radiology* 35 (1917): 379.

40. "Dr. Frank Butler Granger," *Physical Therapeutics* 46 (1928): 557–568.

41. *The Medical Department of the U.S. Army in the World War* XIII: 6.

42. *American Journal of Electro-Therapeutics and Radiology* 35 (1917): 481–482.

43. *JAMA* 69 (1917): 1524–1525.

44. *New York Times*, September 17, 1917, p. 1.

45. *Joint Committee on Education and Labor, April 30–May 2, 1918* (S.4284, H.R. 11367, 65th Congress, 2d Session), p. 71.

46. Senate Document No. 166, *Vocational Rehabilitation of Disabled*

Soldiers and Sailors (Washington, D.C.: U.S. Government Printing Office, 1918).

47. Ibid., pp. 16–26.
48. Ibid., pp. 26–29.
49. Ibid., pp. 73–76.
50. Senate Document No. 166.
51. Ibid., pp. 5–16.
52. Ibid., pp. 26–29.
53. *The Medical Department of the U.S. Army in the World War* I: 475.
54. Senate Document No. 173, *Rehabilitation and Vocational Reeducation of Crippled Soldiers and Sailors* (Washington, D.C.: U.S. Government Printing Office, 1918), pp. 38–42.
55. *Joint Committee on Education and Labor,* p. 12.
56. Ibid., pp. 64–66.
57. *Congressional Record,* vol. 56, 65th Congress, 2d Session, 1918, p. 6955.
58. Ibid., p. 7079.
59. Ibid., p. 6958.
60. Ibid., p. 6961.
61. Ibid., p. 7079.
62. *The Medical Department of the U.S. Army in the World War* I: 475–476.
63. Ibid., p. 476.
64. *American Journal of Electro-Therapeutics and Radiology* 36 (1918): 233–236.
65. "After Meat, Mustard," *American Journal of Electro-Therapeutics and Radiology* 35 (1917): 189–190.
66. "Why the Government Delay in Recognition?" *American Journal of Electro-Therapeutics and Radiology* 37 (1919): 232–233.
67. Mildred O. Elson, "The Legacy of Mary McMillan," *Physical Therapy* 44 (1964): 1067–1072.
68. Rosemary Stevens, *American Medicine and the Public Interest* (New Haven: Yale University Press, 1971), pp. 134–135 fn.
69. *Journal of Advanced Therapeutics* 24 (1906): 66–67.
70. Ida Hazenhyer, "A History of the American Physiotherapy Association," *Physiotherapy Review* 26 (1946): 4.
71. "Schools of Physical Education for Reconstruction Aides and the Medical Profession," *JAMA* 70 (1918): 1881–1882.
72. John Bryant, *Convalescence* (New York: The Sturgis Fund of the Burke Foundation, 1927), p. 155.
73. Hazenhyer, "A History of the American Physiotherapy Association," p. 4.
74. "Physio-Therapy's Part in Reconstruction," *Carry On* 1 (1919): 7.
75. Hazenhyer, "A History of the American Physiotherapy Association," p. 3.
76. Elson, "The Legacy of Mary McMillan," pp. 1–4.

77. American Occupational Therapy Association, *Then and Now* (Washington, D.C., 1967), p. 2.

78. Helen L. Hopkins and Helen D. Smith, *Williard and Spackman's Occupational Therapy* (New York: J. B. Lippincott Co., 1978), pp. 4–6.

79. Harriet Heitlinger Woodside, "The Development of Occupational Therapy 1910–1929," *American Journal of Occupational Therapy* 35 (1971): 7–10.

80. Sidney Licht, "The Founding and Founders of the American Occupational Therapy Association," *Occupational Therapy* 21 (1967): 269–276.

81. See, for example, William Rush Dunton, Jr., "Occupation as a Therapeutic Measure," *Medical Record* 83 (1913): 388–389; and "History of Occupational Therapy," *Modern Hospital* 8 (1917): 380–381.

82. *Constitution of the National Society for the Promotion of Occupational Therapy* (Baltimore: Sheppard Hospital Press, 1917), p. 1.

83. Woodside, "The Development of Occupational Therapy 1910–1929," p. 229.

84. William Rush Dunton, Jr., *Prescribing Occupational Therapy* (Springfield, Ill.: Charles C Thomas, 1928), p. 10.

85. "Presidents of the American Occupational Therapy Association (1917–1967)," *American Journal of Occupational Therapy* 21 (1967): 290.

86. Ibid.

87. AOTA, *Then and Now*, pp. 6–7.

88. C. D. Myers, "Pioneer Occupational Therapists in World War I," *American Journal of Occupational Therapy* 2 (1948): 210.

89. "Occupational Aides," *Maryland Psychiatric Quarterly* 8 (1918): 27–28.

90. Margaret A. Neall, "Philadelphia School for Occupational Therapy," *The Annals* 80 (1918): 58–61.

91. Woodside, "The Development of Occupational Therapy 1910–1929," p. 229.

92. *Proceedings of the Second Annual Meeting*, 1918; reprinted in AOTA, *Then and Now*, p. 22.

93. Senate Document No. 166, p. 25.

94. Charles Hanson Toune, "To Our Disabled Soldiers," *Carry On* 1 (1919): 7.

95. Harry Eaton Stewart, "The Reconstruction Program of the United States Public Health Service," *American Journal of Electro-Therapeutics and Radiology* 38 (1920): 205–206; and Curtis E. Lakeman, "Social After-Care of Crippled Soldiers," *American Journal of Care for Cripples* 6 (1918): 11–16.

96. William Seaman Bainbridge, "The Importance of Physical Therapy in Military and Civil Practice," *Military Surgeon* 45 (1919): 663–678.

97. "The Field of Physical Therapy," *New York Medical Journal* 109 (1919): 1132.

98. Frederick Peterson, "Credulity and Cures," *JAMA* 73 (1919): 1739.

99. "Christmas and the Nations at Peace," *American Journal of Nursing* 19 (1918): 154; "Red Cross Nursing Survey," ibid. 19 (1919): 261, 331–332.

100. *The Medical Department of the U.S. Army in the World War* II: 430.

101. *The Medical Department of the U.S. Army in the World War* XIII: 181–187.

4: Foundations for a Division of Labor, 1920–1941

1. Rosemary Stevens, *American Medicine and the Public Interest* (New Haven: Yale University Press, 1971), chaps. 8, 10.

2. *Archives of Physical Therapy, X-Ray, Radium* 7 (1926): 175; and Henry H. Kessler, "Rehabilitation of the Physically Handicapped," *Archives of Physical Therapy* 19 (1938): 753.

3. Paul A. Nelson, "History of the Archives—A Journal of Ideas and History," *Archives of Physical Medicine and Rehabilitation: Cumulative Index, 1920–1969* (American Congress of Rehabilitation Medicine, 1970), pp. 4–22; and Walter J. Zeiter, "The History of the American Congress of Physical Medicine and Rehabilitation," *Archives of Physical Medicine and Rehabilitation* 35 (1954): 683–686.

4. Nelson, "History of the Archives," p. 10.

5. Morris Fishbein, "Council of Physical Therapy," *Archives of Physical Therapy, X-Ray, Radium* 7 (1926): 358.

6. Ibid., p. 356.

7. "Report of the Committee on Present Status of Physical Therapy," *JAMA* 87 (1926): 1302–1303.

8. "Should Physical Therapy Be Hospital Controlled," *Archives of Physical Therapy, X-Ray, Radium* 9 (1928): 507.

9. "Commercializing Physiotherapy," *Archives of Physical Therapy, X-Ray, Radium* 11 (1930): 135.

10. John S. Hibben, "Progress of Physical Therapy," *Archives of Physical Therapy, X-Ray, Radium* 17 (1936): 48.

11. Howard A. Carter, "Council on Physical Therapy," *Archives of Physical Therapy, X-Ray, Radium* 17 (1936): 237.

12. "Report of the Committee on the Present Status of Physical Therapy," *JAMA* 97 (1936): 585.

13. *Archives of Physical Therapy* 22 (1941): 175–176.

14. *Archives of Physical Therapy* 21 (1940): 625.

15. "Registry of Technicians—A Pressing Problem," *Archives of Physical Therapy, X-Ray, Radium* 15 (1934): 241.

16. *JAMA* 87 (1926): 1303.

17. "The Future of Physical Therapy," *Archives of Physical Therapy, X-Ray, Radium* 8 (1927): 87.

18. *JAMA* 107 (1936): 586.

19. Ida Hazenhyer, "A History of the American Physiotherapy Association," *Physiotherapy Review* 26 (1946): 123–126.

20. Richard Kovacs, "The Relation of a Physiotherapy Clinic to Other Departments in Modern Hospitals." Paper read before 32d annual meeting of the American Electro-Therapeutic Association, September 1922, pp. 5–6.

21. Sterling Brinkley, Rehabilitation Medicine Research Unit, Rehabilitation Services Administration, personal communication, April 16, 1974.

22. *Archives of Physical Therapy* 21 (1940): 523.

23. Frank H. Krusen, "The Contributions of Physical Therapy to Medicine," *Archives of Physical Therapy* 9 (1938): 599–600.

24. *Archives of Physical Therapy* 20 (1939): 605; and Nelson, "History of the Archives," p. 23.

25. Russell J. N. Dean, *New Life for Millions: Rehabilitation for America's Disabled* (New York: Hastings House Publishers, 1972), p. 42.

26. Edgar Bick, *Source Book of Orthopedics* (New York: Hafner Publishing Co., 1968), p. 470; and Troy Bagwell, "Physical Therapy in Relation to Orthopedics," *Archives of Physical Therapy* 21 (1940): 684–687.

27. *Military Surgeon* 107 (1950): 427–428.

28. Hazenhyer, "A History of the American Physiotherapy Association," p. 6.

29. *Physiotherapy Review* 9 (1929): 97.

30. Gertrude Beard, "President's Message," *Physiotherapy Review* 7 (June 1927): 3.

31. Hazenhyer, "A History of the American Physiotherapy Association," p. 7.

32. "The American Physiotherapy Association," *Physiotherapy Review* 13 (1933): 226–227.

33. "What's in a Name?" *Physiotherapy Review* 9 (1929): 97.

34. "Extra! Extra! All About the Convention," *Physiotherapy Review* 7 (June 1927): 7.

35. "Annual Report of the Legislative Committee," *Physiotherapy Review* 9 (1929): 157.

36. Hazenhyer, "A History of the American Physiotherapy Association," p. 126.

37. Ibid., pp. 69–71.

38. Ibid., p. 69 (emphasis added).

39. Ibid., p. 124.

40. Julia Tuggle, "What Is a Physiotherapist?" *Physiotherapy Review* 11 (1931): 13.

41. *Physiotherapy Review* 12 (1932): 83.

42. *Physiotherapy Review* 13 (1933): 226.

43. Ibid., pp. 126–127; and *Memorandum*, November 10, 1933, APTA Files.

44. O. N. Andersen, "Educational Standards for Physical Therapy Technicians," *Archives of Physical Therapy, X-Ray, Radium* 17 (1936): 616.

45. Nelson, "History of the Archives," p. 14.

46. Marion G. Smith, "The American Registry of Physical Therapy Technicians," *Archives of Physical Therapy, X-Ray, Radium* 17 (1936): 620.

47. *Memorandum,* May 26, 1934, American Physical Therapy Association Files.

48. Zeiter, "The History of the American Congress of Physical Medicine and Rehabilitation," p. 685.

49. *Physiotherapy Review* 18 (1938): 201–202.

50. Smith, "The American Registry of Physical Therapy Technicians," p. 620.

51. See, for example, "Report of the Representative Serving on the Advisory Board of the American Registry of Physical Therapy Technicians," *Physiotherapy Review* 20 (1940): 234–235.

52. Eliot Freidson, "Professions and the Occupational Principle," in *Professions and Their Prospects,* ed. Freidson (Beverly Hills: Sage Publications, 1973), pp. 19–38.

53. *Memorandum,* November 10, 1933, American Physical Therapy Association Files.

54. Eloise T. Landis, "Does a Physical Therapy Department Contribute to a Hospital," *Physiotherapy Review* 18 (1938): 180.

55. *Physiotherapy Review* 20 (1940): 268–270.

56. *Physiotherapy Review* 18 (1938): 201–202.

57. *Archives of Occupational Therapy* 1 (1922): 71.

58. *Then and Now* (Washington, D.C.: American Occupational Therapy Association, 1967), p. 10.

59. "The Fifth Annual Meeting of the National Society for the Promotion of Occupational Therapy," *Archives of Occupational Therapy* 1 (1922): 145.

60. Ibid., p. 146.

61. *Archives of Occupational Therapy* 1 (1922): 499.

62. *Archives of Occupational Therapy* 21 (1923): 62.

63. Nell Green, "Occupational Therapy for Orthopedic Cases," *Archives of Occupational Therapy* 1 (1922): 269–278.

64. *Then and Now,* p. 10; *Archives of Occupational Therapy* 1 (1922): 164; and *Archives of Occupational Therapy and Rehabilitation* 10 (1931): 13–14.

65. *Archives of Occupational Therapy* 1 (1922): 500.

66. "Thomas Bessell Kidner," *Occupational Therapy and Rehabilitation* 11 (1932): 321–323.

67. *Archives of Occupational Therapy and Rehabilitation* 4 (1925): 227–229, 296.

68. "President's Address," Thomas Bessell Kidner, *Archives of Occupational Therapy* 2 (1923): 423–424.

69. *American Journal of Occupational Therapy* 25 (1971): 1–6.

70. Everett S. Elwood, "The National Board of Medical Examiners and Medical Education, and the Possible Effect of the Board's Program on the Spread of Occupational Therapy," *Occupational Therapy and Rehabilitation* 6 (1927): 341–342.

71. *Archives of Occupational Therapy and Rehabilitation* 14 (1935): 299.

72. "Minimum Standards for Courses of Training in Occupational Therapy," *Archives of Occupational Therapy* 3 (1924): 295–298; and "Report of Committee on Registration," *Occupational Therapy and Rehabilitation* 6 (1927): 58–64.

73. *Occupational Therapy and Rehabilitation* 6 (1927): 410.

74. "The American Hospital Association," *Occupational Therapy and Rehabilitation* 11 (1932): 461.

75. "Solidarity," *Archives of Occupational Therapy* 3 (1924): 75.

76. "Presidents of the American Occupational Therapy Association, 1917–1967," *American Journal of Occupational Therapy* 21 (1967): 292–294.

77. Emily J. Hicks, "A Crusade for Safer Nursing," *American Journal of Nursing* 38 (1938): 7–8.

78. "New York State Nurses," *Occupational Therapy and Rehabilitation* 17 (1938): 203–204.

79. T. B. Kidner, "Occupational Therapy, Its Development and Possibilities," *Archives of Occupational Therapy and Rehabilitation* 10 (1931): 7–8.

80. "Occupational Therapy in Its Relationship to Physiotherapy," *Physiotherapy Review* 12 (1932): 146.

81. Martha R. Emig, "Correlation of Physiotherapy to Occupational Therapy," *Physiotherapy Review* 8 (August 1928): 50.

82. Caroline N. Shaw, "Occupational Therapy," *Physiotherapy Review* 7 (December 1927): 34.

83. Kidner, "Occupational Therapy, Its Development and Possibilities," pp. 7–8; *Archives of Occupational Therapy and Rehabilitation* 14 (1935): 197; and *Physiotherapy Review* 17 (1937): 136–137.

84. Eleanor Clarke Slagle, "To Organize an 'O.T.' Department," *Occupational Therapy and Rehabilitation* 6 (1927): 125.

85. Philip Smith, "Relation Between Social Service and Occupational Therapy," *Occupational Therapy and Rehabilitation* 14 (1935): 102.

86. Ibid. p. 103.

87. Lucy G. Morse, "Should the Nurse or the Occupational Ther-

apist Offer Diversion in a General Hospital?" *Occupational Therapy and Rehabilitation* 16 (1937): 160.

88. "Nursing and Occupational Therapy," *Occupational Therapy and Rehabilitation* 18 (1939): 64.

89. Alice H. Dean, "The Volunteer Worker," *Occupational Therapy and Rehabilitation* 6 (1927): 209.

90. Frank Krusen, "The Relationship of Physical Therapy and Occupational Therapy," *Archives of Occupational Therapy and Rehabilitation* 13 (1934): 69–76.

91. "Physiotherapy or Psychotherapy," *Occupational Therapy and Rehabilitation* 10 (1931): 123.

92. John Coulter, "Necessity of Medical Supervision in Occupational Therapy," *Archives of Occupational Therapy and Rehabilitation* 10 (1931): 19–23; and "Report of the Committee on the Present Status of Physical Therapy," *JAMA* 107 (1936): 584–587.

93. *Archives of Occupational Therapy and Rehabilitation* 17 (1938): 193, 355.

94. Ibid.

5: The Rediscovery of Rehabilitation, 1941–1950

1. Frank Krusen, "The Contributions of Physical Therapy to Medicine," *Archives of Physical Therapy* 19 (1938): 597.

2. Ibid., p. 598.

3. Ibid., pp. 599–601.

4. Ibid., pp. 599–600.

5. "Physical Therapy in the Next War," *Archives of Physical Therapy* 19 (1938): 432–433.

6. William H. Schmidt, "Open Letter to the Surgeon General of the United States Army by the President of Our Congress," *Archives of Physical Therapy* 21 (1940): 367.

7. "Has the War Preparedness Committee Forgotten Physical Therapy?" *Archives of Physical Therapy* 21 (1940): 425–427.

8. Paul H. Nelson, "The American Congress of Rehabilitation Medicine 1923–1973. Fifty Years of Progress," *50th Anniversary Program* (Chicago: American Congress of Rehabilitative Medicine, 1973), p. 7.

9. "The Need for Physicians Trained in Physical Therapy for the Army," *Archives of Physical Therapy* 23 (1942): 109.

10. "Present Status of Treatment of Poliomyelitis," *Archives of Physical Therapy* 23 (1942): 44.

11. "The Kenny Treatment for Poliomyelitis," *Archives of Physical Therapy* 23 (1942): 367.

12. Frank Krusen, "The Place of Physical Medicine in the Defense Program," *Archives of Physical Therapy* 23 (1942): 453–495.

13. Ibid., p. 453.

14. Howard A. Rusk, *A World to Care For: The Autobiography of Howard A. Rusk* (New York: Random House, 1972).

15. Paul D. Magnuson, *Ring the Night Bell* (Boston: Little, Brown and Co., 1960): p. 195.

16. Rusk, *A World to Care For*, pp. 12–21.

17. *U.S. Army in World War II: The Medical Department: Hospitalization and Evacuation, Zone of the Interior* (Washington, D.C.: Office of the Chief of Military History, 1956), pp. 117–118; *The Medical Department, U.S. Army in World War II: Organization and Administration in World War II* (Washington, D.C.: Office of the Surgeon General, 1963), pp. 213–214; and Rusk, *A World to Care For*, pp. 86–90.

18. Russell J. N. Dean, *New Life for Millions: Rehabilitation for America's Disabled* (New York: Hastings House Publishers, 1972), p. 73.

19. Esco Obermann, *A History of Vocational Rehabilitation in America* (Minneapolis: T. S. Denison and Co., 1965), pp. 279–290.

20. Dean, *New Life for Millions*, pp. 78–79.

21. Obermann, *A History of Vocational Rehabilitation*, pp. 274–290.

22. *The Medical Department*, pp. 213–214.

23. C. Warren Bledsoe, "From Valley Forge to Hines: Truth Old Enough to Tell," American Association of Workers for the Blind, Inc. (reprint from *Blindness*, 1969).

24. *U.S. Army in World War II*, pp. 119–120, 189–190.

25. Ibid., pp. 189–190; *The Medical Department*, p. 214; and Rusk, *A World to Care For*, pp. 89–90.

26. See, e.g., the following articles in the *Archives of Physical Therapy*: "A New Specialty of Physical Medicine," 24 (1943): 682; "The Future Development of Physical Medicine," 25 (1944): 455–460; "New Horizons in Physical Medicine," 25 (1944): 525–528; and "Physical Medicine Comes into Its Own," 25 (1944): 721.

27. "Physical Therapy in Education and Research," *Archives of Physical Therapy* 22 (1941): 619–620.

28. Fred B. Moor, "The Future of Physical Medicine," *Archives of Physical Therapy* 23 (1942): 588–591.

29. *Report of the Baruch Committee on Physical Medicine*, April 1944, p. 1.

30. Ibid., p. 2.

31. Ibid., pp. 3–14.

32. Ibid., p. 42.

33. Ibid., pp. 2, 42–48.

34. Ibid., pp. 2–4; and *Journal of Rehabilitation* 11 (1945): 30.

35. Ibid., pp. 94–95.

36. Ibid., pp. 56–57.

37. *Annual Report of the Baruch Committee on Physical Medicine*, April 1, 1944, to March 31, 1945, pp. 6–7, 18.

38. H. Worley Kendell, "An Early Progress Report on the De-

velopment of the Department of Physical Medicine at the University of Illinois College of Medicine," *Archives of Physical Medicine* 28 (1947): 174.

39. Frank H. Krusen, "Historical Development of Physical Medicine and Rehabilitation During the Last Forty Years," *Archives of Physical Medicine and Rehabilitation* 50 (1969): 2–3.

40. Henry B. Gwynn, "Reconditioning in Civilian Hospitals," *Archives of Physical Medicine* 26 (1945): 276; and "Reconditioning of Civilian Patients," *Archives of Physical Medicine* 26 (1945): 300.

41. Robert Elman, "Physical Medicine in Surgical Convalescence," *Archives of Physical Medicine* 27 (1946): 197.

42. "Early Mobilization in the Postoperative Care of Surgical Patients," *Archives of Physical Medicine* 27 (1946): 513.

43. "The Baruch Committee on Physical Medicine," *Journal of Rehabilitation* 11 (March 1945): 32.

44. Ibid., p. 31.

45. "A New Specialty of Physical Medicine," *Archives of Physical Therapy* 24 (1943): 682.

46. Ibid., p. 683.

47. *Archives of Physical Therapy* 25 (1944): 52, 177, 230.

48. "A Memorable Annual Meeting," *Archives of Physical Therapy* 25 (1944): 557–558.

49. "Physical Medicine in the United States," pp. 39–40.

50. Ibid., p. 40.

51. "Physiatrist," *Archives of Physical Medicine* 27 (1946): 287.

52. *Annual Report of the Baruch Committee,* April 1, 1945, to December 31, 1946, p. 3.

53. "American Board of Physical Medicine," *Archives of Physical Medicine* 28 (1947): 531.

54. *Army Medical Specialists' Corps* (Washington, D.C.: Office of the Surgeon General, 1968), pp. 56–59.

55. Ibid., pp. 57, 114–117.

56. Ida May Hazenhyer, "A History of the American Physiotherapy Association," *Physiotherapy Review* 26 (1946): 177 (this quote was an excerpt from an article in *JAMA,* March 11, 1939).

57. Ibid.

58. Ibid., pp. 177–178.

59. Ibid., p. 178.

60. Emma E. Vogel, "The History of Physical Therapists, United States Army," *Fourth Mary McMillan Lecture* (APTA, 1967), p. 9.

61. Hazenhyer, "A History of the American Physiotherapy Association," pp. 175–179; and *Memorandum,* American Physical Therapy Association Files, October 26, 1940, and September 25, 1941.

62. *Memorandum,* APTA Files, October 26, 1940.

63. Rosemary Stevens, *American Medicine and the Public Interest* (New Haven: Yale University Press, 1971), pp. 114, 256, 277–285.

64. Hazenhyer, "A History of the American Physiotherapy Association," pp. 180–181.

65. *Army Medical Specialists' Corps*, pp. 105–106, 114–115; and Hazenhyer, "A History of the American Physiotherapy Association," p. 181.

66. *Army Medical Specialists' Corps*, pp. 114–117, 171–172.

67. Vogel, "The History of Physical Therapists, United States Army," p. 8.

68. Ibid., p. 10.

69. "Recommended Change in Essentials of an Acceptable School for Physical Therapy Technicians," *JAMA* 129 (1945): 463; and *Archives of Physical Medicine* 26 (1945): 659.

70. Hazenhyer, "A History of the American Physiotherapy Association," p. 177.

71. *Memorandum*, APTA Files, December 17, 1947.

72. "Physical Therapy Technicians," *Archives of Physical Therapy* 24 (1943): 408.

73. *Memorandum*, APTA Files, May 17, 1944.

74. Barbara White, Editor, *Physical Therapy* (pers. comm., June 19, 1974); and Vogel, "The History of Physical Therapists, United States Army," p. 11.

75. *Army Medical Specialists' Corps*, pp. 290–291.

76. Jack Hofkosh, Director of Physical Therapy, Institute of Rehabilitation Medicine (pers. comm., November 8, 1974).

77. *Army Medical Specialists' Corps*, p. 287.

78. Hazenhyer, "A History of the American Physiotherapy Association," pp. 177–178.

79. *Memorandum*, APTA Files, November 1, 1945.

80. *Army Medical Specialists' Corps*, pp. 4, 85–93; and *U.S. Army in World War II*, p. 251.

81. *Army Medical Specialists' Corps*, pp. 6–7, 101–102.

82. Cf. pp. 101–103.

83. *Army Medical Specialists' Corps*, pp. 104–105; *American Occupational Therapy Newsletter* 3 (November 1941): 1; and 5 (July 1943): 2.

84. *American Occupational Therapy Newsletter* 3 (March 1942): 2.

85. *Army Medical Specialists' Corps*, p. 105.

86. Ibid., p. 102.

87. Ibid., pp. 103–104.

88. *American Occupational Therapy Newsletter* 5 (July 1943): 2; and 6 (May 1944): 2.

89. *Army Medical Specialists' Corps*, p. 172.

90. Ibid., pp. 106–107, 287.

91. *American Occupational Therapy Newsletter* 6 (August 6, 1944): 2.

92. *U.S. Army in World War II*, p. 252.

93. *Report of the Baruch Committee on Physical Medicine*, April 1944, pp. 53, 77.

94. "Occupational Therapy a Part of Physical Medicine," *Archives of Physical Therapy* 25 (1944): 230.

95. Wilma West, Former President, AOTA (personal communication, June 25, 1974).

96. Anne Cronin Mosey, "Involvement in the Rehabilitation Movement—1942–1960," *American Journal of Occupational Therapy* 25 (1971): 235.

97. T. Arthur Turner, "The Relationship of Public and Private Agencies," *Journal of Rehabilitation* 11 (March 1945): 17.

98. "Physical Medicine Service Established in Army Hospitals of More than 750 Beds," *Archives of Physical Medicine* 28 (1947): 47.

99. Benjamin Strickland, "Physical Medicine in the Army," *Archives of Physical Medicine* 28 (1947): 233–234.

100. Alfred Ebel, Physical Medicine Department, Montefiore Hospital (personal communication, March 4, 1974).

101. Strickland, "Physical Medicine in the Army," p. 232.

102. *Army Medical Specialists' Corps*, pp. 135–136.

103. Magnuson, *Ring the Night Bell*, p. 318.

104. Benjamin Wells, Former Deputy Chief Medical Director, Veterans Administration (personal communication, May 20, 1974).

105. Bledsoe, "From Valley Forge to Hines," p. 97; and Dean, *New Life for Millions*, pp. 92–93.

106. *Medical Care of Veterans* (Washington, D.C.: U.S. Government Printing Office, 1967), p. 193.

107. Rusk, *A World to Care For*, p. 91; and Dean, *New Life for Millions*, pp. 92–94.

108. James Garrett, Assistant Administrator of Research and Training, Rehabilitation Services Administration (pers. comm., April 15, 1974); and Donald Covalt, "Physical Medicine and Rehabilitation in the V.A.," *Archives of Physical Medicine* 28 (1947): 327.

109. Magnuson, *Ring the Night Bell*, pp. 278–288.

110. Dean, *New Life for Millions*, pp. 95–96.

111. Magnuson, *Ring the Night Bell*, pp. 323–350.

112. C. Warren Bledsoe, Division for the Blind, Rehabilitation Services Administration (personal communication, April 15, 1974).

113. "Trends in Training in Physical Medicine," *Archives of Physical Medicine* 28 (1947): 301; and Covalt, "Physical Medicine and Rehabilitation in the V.A.," p. 328.

114. William H. Redkey, "Bringing Rehabilitation to the Hospital," *Journal of Rehabilitation* 14 (February 1948): 10–12.

115. H. D. Bowman, "Medical Rehabilitation in the Veterans Administration," unpublished report, March 1972, p. 21.

116. Bledsoe, "From Valley Forge to Hines," p. 125.

117. Bledsoe (personal communication, April 15, 1974); and Donald Blasch, "Orientation and Mobility Fans Out," *Blindness 1971*, pp. 9–10.

118. Florence Linduff Knowles, Former Chief of Physical Therapy, Veterans Administration (personal communication, May 14, 1974).

119. Neil Sheldon, Chief, Speech and Hearing Department, Montefiore Hospital and Medical Center (personal communication, July 24, 1973).

120. *Memorandum,* AMA Files, January 1962.

121. Letter from ASHA to NCA, AMA Files, June 1962.

122. Max Goldstein, "The Otologist and the Speech Pathologist," *Journal of Speech Disorders* 3 (1938): 231; and Sidney Weissman, "Speech Pathology in Medical Colleges," *Journal of Speech Disorders* 3 (1938): 215–216.

123. Bowman, "Medical Rehabilitation in the Veterans Administration," p. 52.

124. *Memorandum,* AMA Files, September 1963 and December 1963.

125. *Report: Physical Medicine and Rehabilitation Service* (unpublished report of Medical Director's Advisory Committee of Hospital Directors, January 1972), p. 2.

126. Warren Smith, Chief, Corrective Therapy, Veterans Administration (personal communication, June 21, 1974).

127. Ibid.; and Hofkosh (personal communication, November 8, 1974).

128. Knowles (personal communication, May 14, 1974).

129. "Trends in Training in Physical Medicine," p. 302.

130. Ibid., p. 301.

131. Ibid., p. 302.

132. Ibid., p. 302; Harry Etter, "Physical Medicine in the Navy," *Archives of Physical Medicine* 28 (1947): 537; and John Coulter, "History and Development of Physical Medicine," ibid., p. 602.

133. Etter, "Physical Medicine in the Navy," p. 537.

134. *Memorandum,* APTA Files, March 6, 1952.

135. *Memorandum,* APTA Files, September, 1953.

136. Howard Rusk (personal communication, November 8, 1974).

137. Smith (personal communication, June 21, 1974).

138. Creston Herold, Executive Director, American Congress of Rehabilitation Medicine (personal communication, July 29, 1974).

139. *Correspondence,* AMA Files, February 15, 1971.

140. Smith (personal communication, June 21, 1974).

141. *Personal Qualifications for Medicare Personnel* (Washington, D.C.: DHEW, 1968), chap. 5.

142. White (personal communication, June 20, 1974).

143. *Report: Physical Medicine and Rehabilitation Service,* p. 3.

144. *Department of Medicine and Surgery Supplement,* M-2, pt. VIII (Washington, D.C.: Veterans Administration, 1966), chap. 4.

145. Knowles (personal communication, May 14, 1974); and Wells (personal communication, May 20, 1974).

146. "Physical Medicine and Rehabilitation," *Archives of Physical Medicine* 30 (1949): 107–108; and "Physical Medicine and Rehabilitation at the Annual Meeting of the American Medical Association," ibid., p. 459.

147. Ibid., pp. 533, 595.

148. See, e.g., Howard Rusk, "The Broadening Horizons of Rehabilitation and Physical Medicine," *Archives of Physical Medicine*, 30 (1949), 26–28; and Otto Eisert, "Rehabilitation of the Chronically Medically Ill," ibid., p. 441.

149. James Folsom, Medical Director, Physical Medicine and Rehabilitation, Veterans Administration (personal communication, May 20, 1974).

150. *Memorandum*, APTA Files, April 15, 1949; December 3, 1949.

151. *Model Law*, APTA Files, November 1950.

152. Cf. pp. 115–117.

153. *Memorandum*, APTA Files, April 15, 1949.

154. Ibid., January 1951.

155. Ibid., January 1951.

156. Ibid., March 1952.

157. Ibid., September 1951.

158. Ibid., March 1952.

159. *American Occupational Therapy Newsletter* 6 (May 1946): 1.

160. Ibid., 10 (July 1951): 7.

161. Charlotte Bone, "Origin of the American Journal of Occupational Therapy," American Occupational Therapy Association, 1971, pp. 8–10.

162. *American Occupational Therapy Association Newsletter* 11 (August 1952): 8.

163. Ibid., 8 (November 1949): 2.

164. Mosey, "Involvement in the Rehabilitation Movement—1942–1960," p. 235.

6: The Redivision of Labor, 1950–1980

1. Editorial, *Physical Therapy Review* 31 (1951): 194; and Barbara Oak Robinson, "The Physical Therapy Profession and the Political Process," *Physical Therapy Review* 36 (1956): 393.

2. "President's Report, 1950–51," *Physical Therapy Review* 31 (1951): 378–379.

3. Robinson, "The Physical Therapy Profession and the Political Process," p. 396.

4. APTA Files, July 1954.

5. Ibid., "Recommendations for State Laws," 1957.

6. Ibid., "Letter to Dr. Raymond McKeown," 1959.

7. Ibid., May 1958.

8. Ibid., Memorandum (confidential), 1959.

9. Ibid., "Statement for the AMA Joint Committee to Study Para-medical Areas in Relation to Medicine," 1959.

10. *American Journal of Occupational Therapy* 16 (1962): 102.

11. APTA Files, July 1960.

12. Agnes Snyder, Editorial, "Licensure and Independent Prac-tice," *Physical Therapy Review* 40 (1960): 530–531.

13. Ibid., p. 530.

14. Eleanor Flanagan and Helen Kaiser, "The Challenge to Phys-ical Therapy in Present Day Medicine," *Journal of the American Physical Therapy Association* 42 (1962): 402–404.

15. Editorial, "Medical Supervision of Physical Therapy," *Archives of Physical Medicine and Rehabilitation* 34 (1953): 502.

16. Editorial, "Direct Medical Supervision of Physical Therapy," *Archives of Physical Medicine and Rehabilitation* 35 (1954): 99.

17. Ibid., p. 100.

18. Editorial, "Teamwork in Medicine," *Archives of Physical Med-icine and Rehabilitation* 36 (1955): 43–45.

19. Donald L. Rose, "The Practice of Physical Medicine and Rehabilitation," *Archives of Physical Medicine and Rehabilitation* 40 (1959): 3.

20. Ibid., p. 4.

21. Joseph G. Benton, "Physical Medicine and Rehabilitation— Retrospect and Prospect," *Archives of Physical Medicine and Rehabili-tation* 44 (1963): 150.

22. Editorial, "Medical Direction for Physical Therapy Schools," *Archives of Physical Medicine and Rehabilitation* 41 (1960): 166–168.

23. Patricia Evans, Director of the Department of Educational Affairs, APTA (personal communication, June 19, 1974).

24. Laurence W. Friedmann, "Medicine, Nursing, and Physical Therapy," *Archives of Physical Medicine and Rehabilitation* 52 (1971): 405–406.

25. Katherine A. Sawner, "Physical Therapy, Medicine, and Oc-cupational Therapy," *Archives of Physical Medicine and Rehabilitation* 52 (1971): 409.

26. APTA, "Evolution of Physical Therapy as a Profession and Its Curriculum," APTA, Department of Education, 1982.

27. Ray Siegelman, Executive Director, Massachusetts Chapter, APTA (personal communication, June 22, 1983).

28. Minutes of the Joint Committee of the AHA and APTA, June 4, 1955.

29. Ibid., June 4, 1955; December 2, 1958; January 16, 1959.

30. Ibid., February 21, 1958; December 2, 1958; March 21, 1958.

31. "House Adopts Position Paper on JCAH Standards," *Progress Report* 1 (July 1972): 3.

32. Ibid.

33. "Revised JCAH Standards Implemented," *Progress Report* 1 (May 1972): 5.

34. "House Adopts Position Paper on JCAH," p. 3.

35. Robert C. Bartlett, "The 1977 Presidential Address," *Physical Therapy* 57 (1977): 1251.

36. Charles Magistro, "The 1975 Presidential Address," *Physical Therapy* 55 (1975): 1204–1205.

37. Walter M. Solomon, "The American Congress of Physical Medicine and Rehabilitation: Its Significance and Purpose," *Archives of Physical Medicine and Rehabilitation* 34 (1953): 604.

38. Minutes of the Joint Committee of the AHA and APTA, July 2, 1961.

39. AMA Files, October 1965.

40. Minutes of the Joint Committee of the AHA and APTA, June 22, 1962.

41. Magistro, "The 1975 Presidential Address," p. 1202.

42. Patricia R. Evans, "Accreditation—Vehicle for Change, Part II," *Physical Therapy* 58 (1978): 443.

43. AMA Files, "Meeting of Office of Education, the APTA, and the AMA," December 8, 1972; "Meeting of Representatives of the APTA and AMA Division of Medical Education," January 4, 1973.

44. Magistro, "The 1975 Presidential Address," pp. 1203–1204.

45. Ibid., p. 1203.

46. Grant C. Snarr, Letter to the Editor, *Physical Therapy* 56 (1976): 734.

47. Charles M. Magistro, "The 1976 Presidential Address," *Physical Therapy* 56 (1976): 1235–1236.

48. Bartlett, The 1977 Presidential Address," pp. 1250–1251.

49. Robert C. Bartlett, "The 1978 Presidential Address," *Physical Therapy* 58 (1978): 1329.

50. Helen J. Hislop, "Of Professional Bondage," *Archives of Physical Medicine and Rehabilitation* 59 (1978): 107.

51. *Progress Report* 8 (January 1978): 3.

52. Hislop, "Of Professional Bondage," p. 107; Eugene Michaels, Executive Director, APTA (personal communication, July 5, 1983).

53. *American Journal of Occupational Therapy* 6 (1952): 48.

54. Clare McCarthy, Chief of Physical Therapy, Children's Hospital, Boston (personal communication, June 30, 1983).

55. Jack Hofkosh, Chief of Physical Therapy, Institute of Rehabilitation Medicine (personal communication, November 4, 1974).

56. Beatrice Wade, "From the Study of State Licensure," *American Journal of Occupational Therapy* 14 (1960): 90.

57. Wilma West, Former President, AOTA (personal communication, June 25, 1974).

58. Cordelia Myers, Editor, *American Journal of Occupational Therapy* (personal communication, June 25, 1974).

59. "AOTA Gets Washington Consultant," *American Occupational Therapy Newsletter* 20 (February 1968): 2.

60. Fran Aquaviva, Coordinator of Special Projects, AOTA (personal communication, June 25, 1974).

61. "Full Swing Into Political Action," *Occupational Therapy* 32 (April, 1978): 1.

62. "AOTPAC," *Occupational Therapy* 33 (April 1979): 7.

63. Editorial, *American Journal of Occupational Therapy* 17 (1963): 167.

64. Editorial, *American Journal of Occupational Therapy* 18 (1964): 65.

65. Mildred Sleeper, Guest Editorial, *American Journal of Occupational Therapy* 18 (1964): 114.

66. *American Journal of Occupational Therapy* 27 (1963): 79.

67. Wilma L. West, "The President's Address," *American Journal of Occupational Therapy* 29 (1965): 31–33.

68. Mae D. Hightower-Vandamm, "Presidential Address," *American Journal of Occupational Therapy* 32 (1978): 551–552.

69. Jerry A. Johnson, "Occupational Therapy: A Model for the Future," *American Journal of Occupational Therapy* 27 (1973): 5.

70. Jerry A. Johnson, Nationally Speaking, *American Journal of Occupational Therapy* 28 (1974): 7.

71. Jerry A. Johnson, "Delegate Assembly Address, April 9, 1976," *American Journal of Occupational Therapy* 30 (1976): 447–448.

72. Hightower-Vandamm, "Presidential Address," pp. 551–552.

73. Jay Cocks, "Late, Late Edition," *Time* 104 (December 23, 1974): 4.

74. "Spotlight on OT," *Occupational Therapy* 29 (February 1975): 1.

75. *American Journal of Occupational Therapy* 33 (1979): 787.

76. Anne Cronin Mosey, "Involvement in the Rehabilitation Movement—1942–1960," *American Journal of Occupational Therapy* 25 (1971): 235.

77. Ibid.

78. Johnson, "Occupational Therapy: A Model for the Future," p. 1.

79. Hightower-Vandamm, "Presidential Address," p. 552.

80. June Mazer and Wells Goodrich, "The Prescription: An Anachronistic Procedure in Psychiatric Occupational Therapy," *American Journal of Occupational Therapy* 12 (Pt. I, 1958): 165–170.

81. Vernon L. Nickel, "The Therapist and the Profession," *Proceedings of the 1960 AOTA Conference.*

82. William R. Conte, "The Occupational Therapist as a Therapist," *American Journal of Occupational Therapy* 14 (1960): 1–3, 12.

83. Gail S. Fidler, "The Prescription in Occupational Therapy," *American Journal of Occupational Therapy* 17 (1983): 122.

84. Ibid., pp. 122–123.

85. Felix Millan, Letter to the Editor, *American Journal of Occupational Therapy* 17 (1963): 209.

86. Jerry A. Johnson, "Mission Alpha: A New Beginning," *American Journal of Occupational Therapy* 31 (1977): 147–148.

87. Jerry A. Johnson, "Commitment to Action," *American Journal of Occupational Therapy* 30 (1976): 137.

88. H. Tristram Engelhardt, Jr., "Defining Occupational Therapy and the Virtues of Occupation," *American Journal of Occupational Therapy* 31 (1977): 666–672.

89. J. Sanbourne Bockoven, "Legacy of Moral Treatment—1800's to 1910," *American Journal of Occupational Therapy* 25 (1971): 224.

90. "Task Force on Target Populations, Report I," *American Journal of Occupational Therapy* 28 (1974): 158–163; and Anne Cronin Mosey, "An Alternative: The Biopsychosocial Model," ibid., p. 139.

91. "Task Force on Target Populations, Report I," p. 163.

92. Mae D. Hightower-Vandamm, "The Far-Reaching Impact of the Renaissance—Occupational Therapy 1979," *American Journal of Occupational Therapy* 33 (1979): 760.

93. "Task Force on Target Populations, Report II," *American Journal of Occupational Therapy* 28 (1974): 234.

94. Frank P. Grad, "Legal Alternatives to Certification," *American Journal of Occupational Therapy* 28 (1974): 39.

95. Cordelia Myers, Editorial, *American Journal of Occupational Therapy* 27 (1973): 343; and Johnson, "Occupational Therapy: A Model for the Future," p. 4.

96. Frank Stein, "Occupational Therapy Services in the Prevention of Illness," *American Journal of Occupational Therapy* 31 (1977): 225–226; Shelly Lane Gammage et al., "The Occupational Therapist and Terminal Illness: Learning to Cope with Death," ibid. 30 (1976): 294–299; Anne G. Morris, "Parent Education in Well-Baby Care: A New Role for the Occupational Therapist," ibid. 32 (1978): 75–76; and "Task Force on Target Populations, Report I," p. 161.

97. June L. Mazer, Letter to the Editor, *American Journal of Occupational Therapy* 18 (1964): 29.

98. Mary Reilly, "Occupational Therapy Can Be One of the Great Ideas of 20th Century Medicine," *American Journal of Occupational Therapy* 16 (1962): 1–9.

99. Nationally Speaking, *American Journal of Occupational Therapy* 23 (1969): 209.

100. Edith Winston, "Motivation for Licensure," *American Journal of Occupational Therapy* 30 (1976): 27–30.

101. Marion W. Crampton, "Licensing of Occupational Therapists," *American Journal of Occupational Therapy* 25 (1971): 207.

102. Caroline R. Brayley, "Mobilization of Membership for Legislative Action," *American Journal of Occupational Therapy* 30 (1976): 31.

103. Edith Winston et al., Letter to the Editor, *American Journal of Occupational Therapy* 28 (1974): 241.

104. Jerry A. Johnson, "Licensure," *American Journal of Occupational Therapy* 29 (1975): 73; and Jerry A. Johnson, "No More Waiting," ibid., p. 519.

105. Wilma West, "Problems in the Licensure of Occupational Therapists," *American Journal of Occupational Therapy* 30 (1976): 42.

106. Johnson, "Mission Alpha: A New Beginning," p. 145.

107. "Testing Waters for Licensure," *Occupational Therapy* 29 (June 1975): 4.

108. Carolyn Manville Baum, "State Licensure for Occupational Therapists," *American Journal of Occupational Therapy* 36 (1982): 430.

109. *American Journal of Occupational Therapy* 28 (1974): 562.

110. Winston et al., Letter to the Editor, p. 241.

111. Johnson, "Delegate Assembly Address, April 9, 1976," p. 445.

112. Johnson, "Commitment to Action," p. 144.

113. *American Journal of Occupational Therapy* 28 (1974): 553.

114. Jerry A. Johnson, Nationally Speaking, *American Journal of Occupational Therapy* 29 (1975): 11.

115. "OT Supported in House Hearings," *Occupational Therapy* 29 (October 1975): 3.

116. "HIAA Supports OT Coverage," *Occupational Therapy* 31 (August 1977): 1.

117. *Occupational Therapy* 32 (June 1978): 1.

118. "Special Report: The Baruch Committee on Physical Medicine and Rehabilitation," *Archives of Physical Medicine and Rehabilitation* 32 (1951): 421–422.

119. Frank Krusen, Editorial, "New Section of Physical Medicine and Rehabilitation of the AMA Is Launched," *Archives of Physical Medicine* 31 (1950): 464.

120. Editorial, "Is Physical Medicine Oversold?" *Archives of Physical Medicine* 33 (1952): 299.

121. Ibid.

122. Howard A. Rusk, "Tomorrow Is Not Yesterday," *Archives of Physical Medicine and Rehabilitation* 47 (1966): 5.

123. George M. Piersol, Editorial, "The Doctor Shortage in Physical Medicine," *American Journal of Physical Medicine* 35 (1956): 8.

124. Donald L. Rose, "The Practice of Physical Medicine and Rehabilitation," *Archives of Physical Medicine and Rehabilitation* 40 (1959): 5.

125. Joseph G. Benton, "Physical Medicine and Rehabilitation— Retrospect and Prospect," *Archives of Physical Medicine and Rehabilitation* 44 (1963): 150–151.

126. President's Committee on Employment of the Handicapped, *National Health Care Policies for the Handicapped. Report to the President by National Health Care Policies for the Handicapped Workers' Group* (Washington, D.C.: The White House, 1978).

127. M. T. Southgate, Editorial, "This Is the Decade that Is," *JAMA* 243 (1980): 2177–2216.

128. William M. Fowler, Jr., "Viability of Physical Medicine and Rehabilitation in the 1980's," *Archives of Physical Medicine and Rehabilitation* 63 (1982): 4.

129. Ibid., p. 8.

130. Piersol, "The Doctor Shortage in Physical Medicine," p. 7; and "Is Physical Medicine Oversold?" p. 300.

131. Piersol, "The Doctor Shortage in Physical Medicine," p. 7.
132. *Directory of Medical Specialists* (Chicago: Marquis, 1949, 1951, 1953, 1957), vols. IV, V, VI, VIII.
133. Donald J. Erikson, "Current Problems and Implications of the Future in Physical Medicine and Rehabilitation," *Archives of Physical Medicine and Rehabilitation* 44 (1963): 76.
134. Henry Wechsler, *Handbook of Medical Specialties* (New York: Human Sciences Press, 1976), p. 286.
135. H. J. Lerner, *Manpower Issues and Voluntary Regulation in the Medical Specialty System* (New York: Prodist, 1974), p. 69.
136. E. W. Johnson, "Maturation of a Specialty, Message for the American Board of Physical Medicine and Rehabilitation," *Archives of Physical Medicine and Rehabilitation* 59 (1978): 153–155.
137. Joseph C. Honet, "Diagnosis: A Physiatric Tool for Recruitment," *Archives of Physical Medicine and Rehabilitation* 62 (1981): 6.
138. Frederic J. Kottke, "Future Focus of Rehabilitation Medicine," *Archives of Physical Medicine and Rehabilitation* 61 (1980): 1.
139. *JAMA* 153 (1953): 1552–1553.
140. *Proceedings of the House of Delegates, 1952–1955* (Chicago: AMA, 1958).
141. William Benham Snow, Editorial, "A Message from the President," *Archives of Physical Medicine and Rehabilitation* 34 (1953): 699.
142. William Benham Snow, "The Physiatrist: His Problems, Perceptions and Prospects," *Archives of Physical Medicine and Rehabilitation* 35 (1954): 621.
143. Sidney Licht, Editorial, "Specialty Respectability," *American Journal of Physical Medicine* 35 (1956): 204.
144. Ibid.
145. A. R. Shands, Jr., "Responsibility and Research in Orthopedic Surgery," *Journal of Bone and Joint Surgery* 36A (1954): 695.
146. A. R. Shands, Jr., "A Few Remarks on Physical Medicine," *Southern Medical Journal* 54 (1961): 421.
147. J. Vernon Luck, "Orthopedic Surgery—'Shaping It for Permanence or for Ending,'" *Journal of Bone and Joint Surgery* 44A (1962): 391–392.
148. Licht, "Specialty Respectability," p. 204.
149. Shands, "A Few Remarks on Physical Medicine," p. 425.
150. Erikson, "Current Problems and Implications of the Future of Physical Medicine and Rehabilitation," p. 76.
151. Ibid.
152. Verne T. Inman, "Specialization and the Physiatrist," *Archives of Physical Medicine and Rehabilitation* 47 (1966): 765.
153. A. R. Shands, Jr., "The Attitude of the Physician Toward Rehabilitation," *Journal of Bone and Joint Surgery* 37A (1955): 371.
154. Shands, "A Few Remarks on Physical Medicine," p. 422.
155. Ibid.
156. Inman, "Specialization and the Physiatrist," p. 769.

157. Edward W. Lowman, "The Shadow of a Man," *Archives of Physical Medicine and Rehabilitation* 48 (1967): 502.

158. G. Keith Stillwell, "Meeting a Need," *Archives of Physical Medicine and Rehabilitation* 50 (1969): 489.

159. Inman, "Specialization and the Physiatrist," p. 770.

160. Lowman, "The Shadow of a Man," p. 502.

161. Inman, "Specialization and the Physiatrist," p. 770.

162. Commission on Education in Physical Medicine and Rehabilitation, *Rehabilitation Medicine in American Colleges: Recommendations for Teaching Programs*, Bulletin No. 8, Minneapolis, Minn.

163. Commission on Education in Physical Medicine and Rehabilitation, *The Vocational Interests, Values, and Career Developments of Specialists in Physical Medicine and Rehabilitation*, Bulletin No. 9, Minneapolis, Minn.

164. Douglas A. Fenderson, "The Basis of Physical Medicine and Rehabilitation as a Medical Specialty," *Archives of Physical Medicine and Rehabilitation* 50 (1969): 63.

165. Joseph Goodgold, "Rehabilitation Medicine: Affirmations and Actions," *Archives of Physical Medicine and Rehabilitation* 61 (1980): 8.

166. Friedman, "Medicine, Nursing, and Physical Therapy," p. 405.

167. Ibid.

168. George H. Koepke, "The American Board of Physical Medicine and Rehabilitation: Past, Present and Future," *Archives of Physical Medicine and Rehabilitation* 53 (1972): 11.

169. Donald L. Rose, "A Second Look: Eleventh John Stanley Coulter Memorial Lecture," *Archives of Physical Medicine and Rehabilitation* 43 (1962): 211–212.

170. Lerner, *Manpower Issues and Voluntary Regulation in the Medical Specialty System*, p. 71.

171. Edward E. Gordon, "Of Species and Specialties," *Archives of Physical Medicine and Rehabilitation* 62 (1981): 9.

172. Goodgold, "Rehabilitation Medicine: Affirmations and Actions," p. 9.

173. May L. Watrons, Lorenzo Marcolin, Letters to the Editor, "Hiring Practices of Physicians," *Physical Therapy* 56 (1976): 1286–1287.

174. Donald L. Hiltz, Letter to the Editor, "More on Hiring of Physical Therapists," *Physical Therapy* 56 (1976): 1286–1287; and Alan Leventhol, Letter to the Editor, "More About Physicians Hiring Physical Therapists," ibid. 57 (1977): 305–306.

175. Goodgold, "Rehabilitation Medicine: Affirmations and Actions," p. 9.

176. Ibid.

177. George Coggeshall, Instructor, Department of Physical Therapy, Northeastern University (personal communication, May 18, 1983).

178. Harold Dinken, "The Physiatrist in a Private Hospital," *Archives of Physical Medicine and Rehabilitation* 43 (1962): 449; and Editorial, "Fees in Physical Medicine," ibid. 44 (1963), 663.

179. Licht, "Specialty Respectability," pp. 204–205.

180. Ibid., p. 205.

181. AMA, *Clinical Electroneuromyographic Examinations—Resolution 52*, House of Delegates (Chicago: AMA, 1973).

182. AMA, *Clinical Electroneuromyographic Examinations—Resolution 52 as amended*, House of Delegates (Chicago: AMA, 1973).

183. Koepke, "The American Board of Physical Medicine and Rehabilitation," p. 11.

184. Eugene Moskowitz, "The State of the Academy: A Progress Report," *Archives of Physical Medicine and Rehabilitation* 57 (1976): 48.

185. Jacquelin Perry, Editorial, "Should Physical Therapists Do Electromyography? Yes or No," *Physical Therapy* 55 (1975): 475.

186. Stanley D. Siegelman, Letter to the Editor, "Should Physical Therapists Do Electromyography?" *Physical Therapy* 55 (1975): 898.

187. Nancy T. Farina and Robert H. Cress, Letter to the Editor, *Physical Therapy* 55 (1975): 900.

188. Harriet S. Rosen, Letter to the Editor, "Are PTs Assuming Role of Physicians?" *Physical Therapy* 58 (1978): 69–70.

189. Mitchell Tannenbaum, Letter to the Editor, "Is Knowledge Dangerous?" *Physical Therapy* 58 (1978): 624.

190. Lester J. Goetz, Letter to the Editor, "Are PTs Assuming a Passive Role in the Care of Their Patients?" *Physical Therapy* 58 (1978): 624–626.

191. Joseph Goodgold, Letter to the Editor, "The Author Replies," *Archives of Physical Medicine and Rehabilitation* 61 (1980): 333.

192. Ibid.

193. Tommye Pfefferkorn, *APTA 1981 Annual Report* (Washington, D.C.: APTA, 1981), p. 23.

194. Sue O'Sullivan, Assistant Professor, Department of Physical Therapy, Sargent College of Allied Health Professions, Boston University (personal communication, June 27, 1983).

195. "Does the US Need More Physiatrists?" *Progress Report* 11 (June 1982): 19.

196. Ibid.

Epilogue

1. See chap. 3, pp. 41–45.
2. See chap. 4.
3. See chap. 5.
4. See chap. 5, p. 103.
5. See chap. 3, pp. 59–60.
6. June S. Rothberg, ". . . And It Came to Pass," *Archives of Phys-*

ical Medicine and Rehabilitation 60 (1979): 93; and Thomas P. Anderson, "ACRM at the Crossroads: Time for Reexamination and Reflection," *Archives of Physical Medicine and Rehabilitation* 6 (1980): 58.

7. Viola Robins, "The Challenge to the Profession," *Journal of the American Physical Therapy Association* 45 (1965): 118; Helen J. Hislop, "The Not-So-Impossible Dream," *Physical Therapy* 55 (1975): 1078; and Margaret J. Adamson and May Alyce Anderson, "A Study of the Utilization of Occupational Therapy Assistants and Aides," *American Journal of Occupational Therapy* 20 (1966): 75–79.

8. Magali Sarfatti Larson, *The Rise of Professionalism: A Sociological Analysis* (Berkeley, Los Angeles, London: University of California Press, 1977).

9. "From the National Office," *American Journal of Occupational Therapy* 28 (1974): 238.

10. Betty Fellows, Former Chair, Department of Physical Therapy, Northeastern University (personal communication, June 7, 1983).

11. Eugene Michael, Executive Director, APTA (personal communication, July 5, 1983).

12. Harris S. Cohen and Lawrence H. Miike, *Developments in Health Manpower Licensure: A Follow-up to the 1971 Report on Licensure and Related Health Personnel Credentialing* (Washington, D.C.: U.S. Department of Health, Education, and Welfare, 1973).

13. Ibid., pp. 2–3.

14. Malcolm C. Todd, "Future Directions for Licensure, Certification and Reviewing Performance," in *The Changing Role of the Public and Private Sectors in Health Care* (Report of the 1973 National Health Forum) (New York: National Health Council, 1973), pp. 117–119.

15. Maryland Y. Pennell et al., *Accreditation and Certification in Relation to Allied Health Manpower* (Washington, D.C.: U.S. Department of Health, Education, and Welfare, 1971), p. 11.

16. Robert Alford, *Health Care Politics: Ideological and Interest Group Reform* (Chicago: University of Chicago Press, 1975).

Index

Accreditation, 132–134, 166–167
Activity therapy, 140–142
Advisory board for Medical
   Specialties, 62, 69
Allied Health Act, 123
Allied occupations: assistants,
   166; autonomy of, 123 ff.,
   165–166; competition among,
   103, 114–118, 165; creation of,
   8–9; domination of, 10–11,
   66–70, 72–77, 83–85, 167–169;
   World War II and, 99–108.
   See also Occupational therapy;
   Physical therapy
American Academy of Physical
   Medicine and Rehabilitation,
   131–132, 152, 164
American Association for
   Health, Physical Education
   and Recreation, 101
American Association of
   Electro-Therapeutics and
   Radiology, 45, 58, 63–64, 71
American Association of
   Independent Physical
   Therapists, 127

American Board of
   Rehabilitation Medicine, 99,
   145, 152, 156
American College of Physical
   Therapy, 63
American College of Radiology
   and Physiotherapy, 63
American College of Surgeons,
   77
American Congress of Physical
   Medicine, 98, 116–117, 127,
   131, 132
American Congress of Physical
   Therapy, 63, 64, 94, 98;
   American Registry of
   Physical Therapy
   Technicians, 103, 131;
   occupational therapists and,
   83; physical therapy
   technicians and, 66–69, 76;
   World War II and, 89
American Congress of
   Rehabilitation Medicine, 144,
   164
American Electro-Therapeutic
   Association, 21–22, 27, 30,

American Electro-Therapeutic
Association, (*continued*)
33, 35, 165; Committee on
Affiliation with the AMA, 32;
Committee to Evaluate and
Standardize Apparatus, 37;
Committee on Publicity, 37
American Federation of Labor,
48
American Hospital Association,
77, 80, 83, 129–130, 137, 168
*American Journal of
Electrotherapeutics and
Radiology*, 35
*American Journal of Occupational
Therapy*, 121
American Medical Association:
allied occupations and, 72–
76, 125–126, 132–135, 143,
167–169; corrective therapy
and, 117; Council on Medical
Physics, 149; electrotherapy
and, 34–37; industrial
medicine and, 40; orthopedic
surgery and, 41, 148-149;
physical medicine and, 64,
67, 146, 147, 155–156;
rehabilitation medicine and,
113; specialty definition and,
61–62, 65; War Preparedness
Committee, 89. *See also*
Council on Medical
Education and Hospitals;
Council on Physical Medicine
and Rehabilitation; Physical
Medicine and Rehabilitation
Section
American Occupational
Therapy Association, 167;
Committee on Civil Service
and Legislation, 121;
Committee on Clinical

Practice, 137; Committee on
Occupational Therapy and
National Defense, 105;
commodity definition, 137–
140; founding of, 54–57;
Government Affairs
Department, 136; name
changed, 78; political action,
105, 135–136, 141–145;
Political Action Committee,
136; Public Education
Committee, 105, 121; War
Service Committee, 105, 106
American Orthopedic
Association, 40–41, 150
American Physical Therapy
Association, 167;
Congressional Action
Committee, 136; founding of,
70–71; Interprofessional
Relations Committee, 121;
political action, 100–101, 104,
120–121, 126–135;
relationship to American
Congress of Physical
Therapy, 74–75
American Physiotherapy
Association, 68, 71–75, 77,
100, 102, 104
American Red Cross, 48, 57–58,
91, 102
American Registry of Physical
Therapy, 74–76, 131–132
American Society of Allied
Health Professions, 134, 167
American Society of Physical
Medicine and Rehabilitation,
127, 132
American Speech and Hearing
Association, 113–114
American Women's Physical
Therapy Association, 71

American X-Ray Journal, 31
Apostoli, Georges, 20
Archives of Rehabilitation Medicine, 64
Art therapy, 108, 140, 142
Association of Artificial Limb Manufacturers of the United States, 60
Associations, 174–176

Baruch, Bernard, 94, 109–110
Baruch Committee, 94–97, 107, 110, 145
Beard, George, 19
Blue Cross, 137
Bock, Kenneth, 3
Brackett, Elliott, 41–44
Bradley, Omar, 109–110
Bureau of Health Manpower, 134

Cerebral Palsy Association, 125
Civil Service Commission, 99, 101, 102, 104, 106, 110
Cocks, Jay, 137
Columbia University, 96
Commission on Postsecondary Accreditation, 132–134
Commission on Rehabilitation Medicine, 152
Commodity definition, 7–8, 22, 137–140, 143–145
Community Chest, 121
Competition: between medical and nonmedical groups, 24–25, 32–34, 46–52, 64–66; between medical specialties, 11, 15–16, 31–32, 35, 39–46, 51; between physicians and allied occupations, 10–11, 66–70, 79–80, 153–158. *See also* Occupational therapy,

competitors of; Physical therapy, competitors of
Conference on Occupational Therapy, 106
Conference to Consider Issues in the Accreditation of Allied Health Education, 134
Corbusier, Harold, 70–71
Corrective therapy, 107–109, 112, 115–118, 163, 165
Coulter, John, 91
Council on Medical Education and Hospitals (AMA), 62, 67–68, 73, 119, 146; accreditation of allied schools, 74, 77, 79, 132–134; standards in physical therapy, 100
Council on National Defense, 49, 60
Council on Physical Medicine and Rehabilitation (AMA), 62, 64–67, 73, 74, 76, 98–99, 100, 119, 132, 149
Council on Scientific Assembly, 99
Covalt, Donald, 110
Cross, John B., 18

Dean's committee system, 110
Division of labor: administrative and occupational principles of organization, xiii–xv; boundary determination, 33–34, 76, 159–160; competition in, 10–11, 103; domination and subordination in, 10–11, 72–77, 118–122, 153; Durkheim and, xi, 4–5; market model, xxi–xxii, 7–11; natural growth model, 2–6,

Division of Labor: (continued)
9–10, 13, 159–160; nature of,
xi–xiii; World War I and, 46–
52, 56–60. See also
Competition
Dunton, William, 55, 79
Durkheim, Émile, xi, 4–5

Education therapy, 109, 111
Electromyography, 119, 133,
155–156
Electrotherapy: name change,
39; origins of, 17–26, physical
therapies and, 26–30;
radiology and, 30, 35;
resistance to, 19, 26–27, 34–
36, 58; scientific basis of, 25–
26; specialty status of, 22–23,
30–31, 36. See also Physical
therapy physicians;
Physiotherapy physicians;
Physical medicine

Federal Board for Vocational
Education, 46–52
Federation of Associations for
Cripples, 38
Fragmentation of health care, 1,
2, 167–168
Franklin, Benjamin, 17

Gale, T., 17–18
Garratt, A. C., 18–19
Gilbert, William, 17
Goldthwait, Joel, 41–44, 53
Goode, William, 5
Granger, Frank, 45–46, 51, 53,
71
Gray, Carl, 110

Harvard University, 53
Hawley, Paul, 109

Health Insurance Association of
America, 144
Home Insurance Company, 137
Humphris, Francis Howard, 34

Industrial accidents, 38–39
Industrial physicians, 40
Industrial School for Crippled
and Deformed Children, 42
Industrial therapy, 109
Institute for Rehabilitation
Medicine, 117
Institute for the Crippled and
Disabled, 93
Interdisciplinary Forum, 12
International Association of
Rehabilitation Facilities, 144

Johnson, Jerry, 143–144
Joint Committee on Education
and Labor, 49
Joint Committee on the
Accreditation of Hospitals,
130–131
Journal of Advanced Therapeutics,
27–28
Journal of Electro-Therapeutics, 21

Kellogg Foundation, 101
Kenny, Sister Elizabeth, 90
Kidner, T. B., 78–79, 81
King, William Harvey, 20–24,
27, 29
Knowledge, 2–3, 7–11, 13
Kratzenstein, Christian, 17
Krusen, Frank, 13, 69, 87–88,
90, 110, 146
Kuhn, Thomas, 6

LaFollette and Barden bill, 92
Lambert, Alexander, 38
Larson, Mogali Sarfatti, 7

Licensing legislation, xviii, 16, 33, 117. *See also* Occupational therapy, licensing in; Physical therapy, licensing in

Licht, Sidney, 121

Macgraw, Richard, 3
McMillan, Mary, 71
Magistro, Charles, 133
Magnuson, Paul, 91, 110–111
Manual arts therapy, 109, 111
March of Dimes, 121
Markets: control of, 76–77, 161–169; new, 123, 165–167
Marquette University, 158
Marx, Karl, xii, 6
Massachusetts General Hospital, 26, 41–42, 45
Massage Operators Guild, 66
Massey, George Betton, 21
Medicaid, 123, 128
Medical College of Virginia, 96
Medical Department of the Army, 46–52, 54, 58, 60; Division of Orthopedic Surgery, 41–42, 46, 53; Division of Special Hospitals and Physical Reconstruction, 44, 45, 46, 53
Medical profession, 15–16, 19, 169
Medicare, 123, 128, 136, 143–144
Music therapy, 142

National Association of Licensed Physical Therapists, 127
National Association of Teachers of Speech, 114
National College of Electro-Therapeutics, 24

National Commission on Accreditation, 113, 117, 132
National Council on Rehabilitation, 101
National Easter Seal Society, 121, 143, 144
National Foundation for Infantile Paralysis, 101, 125
National Manufacturers Association, 48
National Research Council, 105–106
National Society for Crippled Children, 122
National Society for the Promotion of Occupational Therapy, 78
National Society of Electro-Therapeutics, 21, 22–23, 27, 30, 165
Neurology, 31–32, 36
New York Medical Practice Act, 102
New York University, 96, 158
Nisbet, Robert, 3, 6
Nurses, 59, 140–141, 162–163

Occupational imperialism, 161–167
Occupational therapy: affiliations, 80; assistants in, 166; competitors of, 82, 107–108, 115, 121–122, 140–143; conflict with physical therapy and, 81–82, 103; focus of, 138–140; licensing in, 81, 135–136, 141–145; marginality of, 165; origins of, 54–57; rehabilitation and, 78–79, 107; rehabilitation medicine and, 83–84, 105–106; relation to physicians, 50, 55, 79–85,

Occupational Therapy:
(*continued*)
105–109, 122, 138–139; self-
certification, 79–81; standards
and training, 104–106; status
of, 121–122; World War II
and, 104–108
*Occupational Therapy and
Rehabilitation*, 121–122
Occupational titles, 173
Office of Education, 133–134
Office of Vocational
Rehabilitation, 93, 112
Orientation and mobility
instructors, 112
Orthopedic surgery:
electrotherapy and, 36;
history of, 40–41; physical
medicine physicians and, 70,
148–153; World War I and,
41–46
Orthotics-Prosthetics, 60, 103,
107–108

Panel on Mental Retardation,
146
Physical medicine: corrective
therapy and, 116–117; decline
of, 146–158; improved status
of, 108–114, 118–119, 145;
marginality of, 165; name
change, 98; orthopedic
surgery and, 148–153;
physical therapy and, 102,
108, 127–131, 153–158;
rehabilitation and, 119;
specialty status of, 99, 163–
164; speech therapy and,
112–114. *See also*
Electrotherapy; Physical
therapy physicians;
Physiotherapy physicians

Physical Medicine and
Rehabilitation Section
(AMA), 145, 149, 155
Physical therapy: assistants in,
166; competitors of, 71–73;
76, 100, 103, 114–118, 165;
conflict with occupational
therapy, 81–82; improved
status of, 101–102, 120, 123–
135; licensing in, 102–103,
120, 124–126, 128–129, 132;
origins of, 45, 51–54, 59, 70–
71; relation to physicians, 54,
67–68, 72–77, 102, 108–109,
153–158; standards in, 99–
100, 104, 158
Physical therapy physicians:
expansion of, 96–97;
improved status of, 64–66;
name change of, 62, 98;
orthopedic surgery and, 89;
rehabilitation and, 94–97; role
in hospitals, 68–70; specialty
status of, 68–70, 87–88, 99;
subordination of allied
occupations, 66–70, 74–77,
83–85; World War II and, 89–
90. *See also* Electrotherapy;
Physical medicine;
Physiotherapy physicians
Physiotherapy physicians:
name change, 39; place in
division of labor, 51–52, 58;
World War I and, 45–46. *See
also* Electrotherapy; Physical
medicine; Physical therapy
physicians; Rehabilitation
medicine
Poliomyelitis, 52, 90
Prehabilitation, 90–91
Private practice, 126–129, 133
Progress, idea of, 2–6

Prudential Insurance Company, 137

Radiological Society, 63
Radiology, 35, 63–64. *See also* X-ray
Reconstruction aides. *See* Occupational therapy, origins of; Physical therapy, origins of
Recreation therapy, 109, 140–141
Red Cross Institute for the Crippled and Disabled, 46
Reed College, 53
Rehabilitation: concept of, xx, 12–13; conflict over, 149–152; physical therapy physicians and, 90–92, 96; reconditioning and, 92–93, 97; Rusk and, 91–94, 96
Rehabilitation medicine. *See* Electrotherapy; Physical therapy physicians; Physiotherapy physicians
Reiser, Stanley, 3
Robarts, Heber, 31
Rockwell, Alphonse, 19
Roentgen Ray Society, 30
Roentgen, Wilhelm, 29
Roosevelt, Eleanor, 94
Rose, Donald, 128
Rusk, Howard, 91–94, 96, 110, 115, 117, 146

Slagle, Eleanor, 55–56
Smith, Adam, xii
Snow, William B., 27
Snow, William B., Jr., 149
Social closures, xiv, xvii
Social work, 108, 140–141

Society of Physical Therapy Physicians, 69
Sorel, Georges, 6
Specialization: causes of, 59–60, 161–169; knowledge and, 7–11; scientific progress and, 2–3; war and, 8–9, 59–60; *See also* Electrotheraphy, specialty status of; Physical therapy physicians, specialty status of
Speech therapy, 60, 109, 112–114, 136
Study of Accreditation of Selected Health Education Programs, 132–134
Surgery, 31, 36, 42, 44

Taggart, Frederick, 3
Technology, xix–xx, 2–3, 8–13, 36–37
Truman, Harry, 110
Tyler, Albert, 63

United States Army, Officer Procurement Service, 102; Physical Medicine Consultants Division, 104, 108
United States Office of Education, 133, 134
United States Public Health Service, 57
University of California, San Francisco, 151
University of Illinois College of Medicine, 96

Veterans Administration, 92–93, 103, 108, 109–118, 154, 169
Veterans' Preference Act, 101
Vocational education, 46–52

214   INDEX

Vocational rehabilitation:
   competition with allied
   occupations, 107–108; laws
   in, 50, 92; medicine and, 46–
   52, 56–57, 92–93; orthopedic
   surgery and, 43

Wadham Committee, 91
Walter Reed Hospital, 53

War Department, 48, 106
War Risk Insurance Act, 47
Weber, Max, xiii, xiv
White House Conference on
   Employment of the
   Handicapped, 146

X-ray, 29–31. *See also* Radiology

COMPARATIVE STUDIES OF HEALTH SYSTEMS AND MEDICAL CARE

General Editor
CHARLES LESLIE

Editorial Board
FRED DUNN, M.D., University of California, San Francisco
RENEE FOX, University of Pennsylvania
ELIOT FREIDSON, New York University
YASUO OTSUKA, M.D., Yokohama City University Medical School
MAGDALENA SOKOLOWSKA, Polish Academy of Sciences
CARL E. TAYLOR, M.D., The Johns Hopkins University
K. N. UDUPA, M.S., F.R.C.S., Banaras Hindu University
PAUL U. UNSCHULD, University of Munich
FRANCIS ZIMMERMANN, Ecole des Hautes Etudes en
Sciences Sociales, Paris

Designer: Robert S. Tinnon
Compositor: Publisher's Typography
Printer: The Murray Printing Company
Binder: The Murray Printing Company
Text: 10/12 Palatino
Display: Palatino